MAGNETIC RESONANCE OF THE MUSCULOSKELETAL SYSTEM

Magnetic Resonance of the Musculoskeletal System

Editor

Thomas H. Berquist, M.D.

Associate Professor
Mayo Medical School; and
Consultant in Diagnostic Radiology
Mayo Clinic, Rochester, Minnesota

Co-Editors

Richard L. Ehman, M.D.

Assistant Professor
Mayo Medical School; and
Associate Consultant
Diagnostic Radiology
Mayo Clinic, Rochester, Minnesota

Michael L. Richardson, M.D.

Assistant Professor
Department of Radiology
University of Washington
School of Medicine
Seattle, Washington

Raven Press ■ New York

Raven Press, 1185 Avenue of the Americas, New York, New York 10036

Made in the United States of America

Library of Congress Cataloging-in-Publication Data

Magnetic resonance of the musculoskeletal system.

    Includes bibliographies and index.
    1. Musculoskeletal system—Diseases—Diagnosis.
2. Magnetic resonance imaging.   I. Berquist, Thomas H.
(Thomas Henry), 1945–   . II. Ehman, Richard L.
III. Richardson, Michael L. [DNLM: 1. Bone Diseases—
diagnosis.   2. Muscular Diseases—diagnosis.
3. Nuclear Magnetic Resonance—diagnostic use.
WE 141 M196]
RC925.7.M34   1986   616.7′0757   85-40577
ISBN 0-88167-220-3

The material contained in this volume was submitted as previously unpublished material, except in the instances in which credit has been given to the source from which some of the illustrative material was derived.

Great care has been taken to maintain the accuracy of the information contained in the volume. However, Raven Press cannot be held responsible for errors or for any consequences arising from the use of the information contained herein.

To my patient family:
my wife, Kay,
and sons, Aric, Matthew, and Andrew

T.H.B.

Preface

The number of clinical magnetic resonance (MR) units is growing rapidly. Software, coil technology, and many hardware developments are evolving. MR imaging has become an accepted clinical tool for evaluating neurological diseases. In general, body imaging has progressed more slowly for a variety of reasons, but musculoskeletal MR is the exception. Musculoskeletal applications of MR are expanding rapidly. Motion artifact is generally not encountered in the extremities. Superior soft tissue contrast and direct coronal and sagittal imaging make MR superior to computed tomography (CT) in many situations. In addition, there is no bone artifact with MR, and nonferromagnetic metal causes less artifact on MR than CT images. Therefore, it is essential for practicing radiologists and clinicians to become aware of the clinical applications of MR in the musculoskeletal system.

The purpose of this volume is to review the principles and applications of MR as they apply to musculoskeletal diseases. The first two chapters, by Nixon and Ehman, provide information on basic principles and how these principles can be applied to provide optimal tissue contrast and characterization. The third chapter, by Berquist, is devoted to patient selection, positioning, and coil techniques. Because MR procedural aspects differ from CT and conventional imaging techniques, it is important to be aware of these factors so that information can be obtained effectively. Factors that affect image quality (coils, number of averages, matrix size, repetition time, etc.), the most commonly used pulse sequences, and patient throughput are thoroughly discussed.

The remaining chapters discuss the applications of MR in specific musculoskeletal diseases. Chapters are pathologically oriented to avoid redundancy. The chapter by Richardson is an exception in that it is devoted to spinal disorders. The final chapter, by Berquist et al., discusses future potential and miscellaneous conditions (areas where MR experience is less extensive). Comparisons of MR with CT, ultrasound, isotopes, and other conventional techniques are emphasized.

Many questions remain unanswered, including optimal field strength and clinical utilization of spectroscopy. Images in this volume demonstrate the use of a variety of radio frequency coils (surface and volume) and field strengths (0.15 to 1.5 tesla).

This volume will be of interest to physicians involved in MR imaging and to clinicians dealing with musculoskeletal diseases who may not be familiar with the principles and applications of MR.

THOMAS H. BERQUIST
RICHARD L. EHMAN
MICHAEL L. RICHARDSON

Acknowledgments

Preparation of this text would not have been possible without the able assistance of our magnetic resonance technologists John Rasmusson, Tim Ruopsa, Kristie Nelson, and Julie Ohm.

We also wish to thank Debbie Roach and Cindy Franke for their diligent effort in preparation of the manuscript. James Martin, Tom Flood, John Hagen, and Vincent Destro were invaluable in the preparation of the images and illustrations.

Finally, we wish to thank the production staff at Raven Press and our editor, Mary Rogers, for assistance in preparation and editing of this text.

Contents

Contributors

Thomas H. Berquist, *Mayo Medical School, and Department of Diagnostic Radiology, Mayo Clinic, Rochester, Minnesota 55905*

Richard L. Ehman, *Mayo Medical School, and Department of Diagnostic Radiology, Mayo Clinic, Rochester, Minnesota 55905*

Clyde A. Helms, *Department of Radiology,. University of California School of Medicine, San Francisco, California 94143*

Harry K. Genant, *Department of Radiology, Medicine, and Orthopedic Surgery, University of California School of Medicine, San Francisco, California 94143*

John R. Nixon, *Mayo Medical School, and Department of Diagnostic Radiology, Mayo Clinic, Rochester, Minnesota 55905*

James A. Rand, *Mayo Medical School, and Department of Orthopedic Surgery, Mayo Clinic, Rochester, Minnesota 55905*

Michael L. Richardson, *Department of Radiology, Harborview Medical Center, University of Washington, Seattle, Washington 98104*

Steven Scott, *Mayo Medical School, and Department of Physical Medicine and Rehabilitation, Mayo Clinic, Rochester, Minnesota 55905*

MAGNETIC RESONANCE OF THE MUSCULOSKELETAL SYSTEM

Basic Principles and Terminology

John R. Nixon

Mayo Medical School, and Department of Diagnostic Radiology,
Mayo Clinic, Rochester, Minnesota 55905

Magnetic resonance (MR) imaging is an exciting new imaging modality that provides excellent soft tissue contrast and spatial resolution. In order to fully utilize the technique, radiologists and other physicians need to have some understanding of the physical principles involved.

Almost all MR imaging systems currently in operation utilize the magnetic properties of the hydrogen nucleus, or proton, in order to create a cross-sectional image. Hydrogen is abundant in biological tissue and gives a relatively strong MR signal compared to other elements such as sodium (^{23}Na) and phosphorus (^{31}P). Hydrogen protons (and other nuclei with an odd number of protons and/or neutrons) possess an inherent spin and a magnetic dipole moment (μ). Normally, the magnetic moments of the individual protons are oriented randomly within a tissue (Fig. 1).

When these protons are placed in a strong stationary magnetic field, designated B_0, they tend to align themselves with the magnetic field. Each proton then behaves like a small gyroscope, and its magnetic moment begins to rotate or precess around the axis of B_0 (usually the Z axis by definition) (Fig. 2). Each proton can exist in one of two energy states. In the low-energy state, the proton's magnetic moment is oriented nearly parallel with the stationary magnetic field. In the high-energy state, the magnetic moment is oriented in the opposite or antiparallel direction relative to B_0. In the resting or equilibrium condition, a slightly greater number of protons exist in the low-energy parallel state than exist in the high-energy antiparallel state. This slight excess, approximately 1 proton per million, produces a net or composite magnetization vector (M) that is oriented in the direction of B_0.

In a uniform magnetic field, all the protons precess at the same rate but are not synchronized in their precession. In other words, they are not precessing in phase with one another, and because of this the vector forces of magnetization perpendicular to B_0 are randomly oriented and cancel out. Therefore, no transverse magnetization exists in this equilibrium state, only longitudinal magnetization in the direction of B_0, resulting from the excess number of low-energy parallel magnetic moments.

1

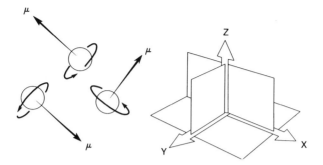

FIG. 1. Hydrogen protons.

The rate at which the protons precess is called the Larmor frequency. This is determined by two factors, the gyromagnetic ratio, which is a constant for the nuclear species involved (e.g., hydrogen), and the strength of the applied magnetic field. Typical MR imaging magnets generate fields between 0.15 and 1.5 T (tesla), depending on the type of system and its operation. These fields are many thousand times stronger than the earth's magnetic field at the surface. Such fields cause hydrogen nuclei to precess at frequencies of 6.4 to 64 MHz, depending directly on the field strength. These frequencies are in the range of radiowaves, so they are called radiofrequency (RF).

Now the MR experiment is about to begin. We can alter the equilibrium state by appling an RF pulse (Fig. 3). The magnetic field component of this pulse is designated B_1 (B_{RF} in the figures). The frequency with which the B_1 pulse alternates is made equal to the Larmor frequency at which the protons are precessing. This RF stimulation causes two things to happen. First, the protons are brought into phase with each other, so that they not only precess at the same frequency, but they also begin to precess in phase. Second, some of the protons in the low-

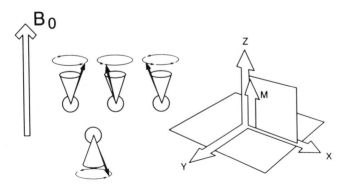

FIG. 2. Precession.

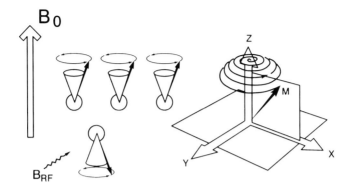

FIG. 3. Resonance.

energy state become excited and enter the high-energy antiparallel state. These two changes cause the net vector M to precess away from its alignment with B_0. The longer the RF pulse is applied, the farther M is tipped, precessing in a large spiral down toward the transverse plane.

These events occur because of resonance. Resonance in a system occurs when a driving force delivers energy at a frequency that matches the inherent frequency of the system. If the RF wave is not of the frequency appropriate for the magnetic field, the Larmor frequency, the hydrogen protons will not resonate. This principle forms the basis of slice selection in cross-sectional imaging.

The longer the protons are stimulated by the applied RF pulse, the more energy they absorb, and a greater number of protons enter the high-energy state. At a certain point, the number of protons in the high-energy state will equal that in the low-energy state, so the vector forces of magnetization that are parallel and antiparallel to B_0 will cancel each other out, and no longitudinal magnetization will be present. Since the individual proton moments are precessing at a slight angle to B_0 and not exactly parallel or antiparallel, and because they are now precessing in phase with each other, the vector forces of magnetization perpendicular to B_0 summate, resulting in a net vector M rotating in the transverse plane. In other words, if the RF pulse is applied long enough or with enough energy, the net M will be tipped by 90° into the transverse (X, Y) plane: A 90° pulse has been applied (Fig. 4).

Alongside the patient are receiver coils made out of copper, each oriented at right angles to the X, Y plane. The vector M rotating in the transverse plane cuts across these coils, and just as a rotating bar magnet would induce a current in a wire coil, M induces a current in the receiver coils. Since the magnetization is rotating at the Larmor frequency, an RF signal is generated (Fig. 5).

Once the RF pulse producing the magnetic field B_1 is turned off, the system returns to equilibrium. The two phenomena that occurred previously when the RF pulse was applied now occur in reverse. The protons dephase, and more return to the low-energy parallel state.

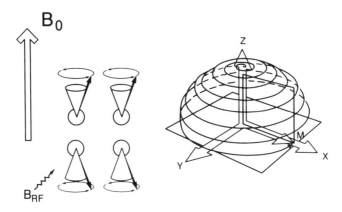

FIG. 4. Resonance.

A measure of the time it takes for dephasing to occur is called T2, or the transverse relaxation time (Fig. 6). Dephasing occurs because each proton is influenced by the local magnetic field created by its neighbor. These local magnetic interactions cause the protons to get out of phase, or relax, in relation to each other. T2 is also called the spin–spin relaxation time, referring to one spinning proton affecting another nearby. Energy is exchanged between protons in the process. Eventually, the individual magnetic moments all become oriented in random directions relative to each other, so the net magnetization in the transverse plane decays to zero as does the MR signal.

Inhomogeneities in an applied magnetic field cause dephasing to occur more rapidly than it would in a perfectly homogeneous field. The rate of transverse

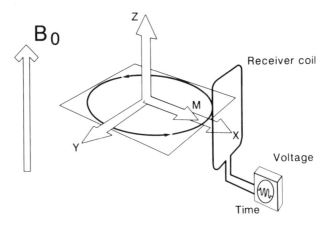

FIG. 5. Radiofrequency signal induced.

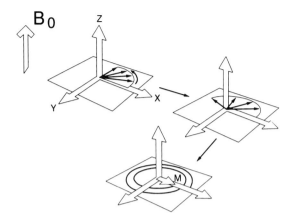

FIG. 6. T2: transverse relaxation; spin–spin relaxation.

relaxation in this setting (such as after a 90° pulse) is described by the term T2 star (T2*) and is determined by a combination of true spin–spin interactions and dephasing due to an inhomogeneous field.

A measure of the time it takes for the protons to reestablish their equilibrium populations in the two different energy states is called T1, or the longitudinal relaxation time. Because it reflects the interaction between the protons and the lattice of their molecular environment, T1 is also called the spin–lattice relaxation time. Energy is given up to the environment by the protons. As more protons relax back to the parallel state, the net magnetization in the direction of the Z axis increases until it reaches the fully relaxed equilibrium state (Fig. 7).

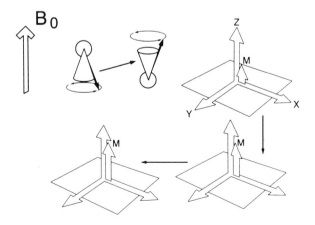

FIG. 7. T1: longitudinal relaxation; spin–lattice relaxation.

T1 is defined as the time it takes for 63% of longitudinal relaxation to occur. In three times T1, 95% of longitudinal relaxation has occurred. In five times T1, essentially 100% has occurred. T2 is defined similarly with regard to transverse relaxation. These relaxation times are important aspects of MR imaging, because different tissues have different relaxation times. These differences give us the contrast between soft tissues in our image and allow us to discriminate pathologic tissue from normal. The reasons for differences in relaxation times and methods of tissue characterization will be discussed further in the next chapter (R. L. Ehman, *this volume*).

A tissue image is created from the signals produced by the precessing protons after they have been stimulated by the RF field B_1. The amplitude of the signals generated depends on the number of precessing protons in a given volume of tissue, referred to as the proton density or spin density, and the relaxation properties of the protons in their various molecular environments, described as T1 and T2. Many soft tissues, whether normal or abnormal, have similar proton densities, so clinical imaging relies mainly on differences in T1 and T2 to provide soft tissue contrast.

Various sequences of RF stimulation are used to obtain images based on these signal parameters. The simplest method might be called repeated free induction decay (FID). This sequence is not often used now in clinical imaging, but it is helpful to understand the principles involved before discussing other more complicated pulse sequences. The repeated FID sequence is just a series of 90° RF pulses, each long enough in duration to tip the proton moments by 90° into the transverse X,Y plane. After each pulse, the precessing protons generate an RF signal in the receiver coils. As dephasing occurs, the magnetization in the transverse plane decays, and the signal dies out. Then as longitudinal relaxation occurs, the magnetization reaccumulates in the Z direction ready to be stimulated again to produce another signal. This process is repeated a number of times, and the signals generated are used to create a tissue image, with the peak amplitude of the signals from the different tissues determining the brightness of the tissue in the image (Figs. 8 and 9).

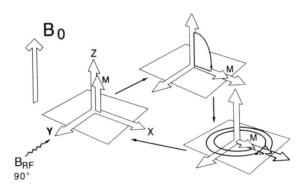

FIG. 8.   Free induction decay.

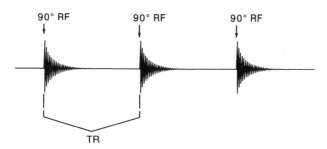

FIG. 9. Free induction decay: proton density, T1; TR $\simeq$ 150–4,000 msec repetition time.

Signal amplitude with the repeated FID sequence is determined by spin density and to some degree by T1, depending on how fast the 90° pulses are repeated. Rapid repetition of the 90° pulses does not give much time for the tissue to relax between pulses. A tissue that has a long T1 relaxation time will not have accumulated much magnetization in the Z direction by the time the next 90° pulse occurs, so little magnetization is available to be flipped into the X, Y plane. Therefore, a weak signal is generated by each successive 90° pulse, and this tissue appears dark in the image. Those tissues that have rapid longitudinal relaxation or short T1 times will accumulate considerable magnetization in the Z direction between pulses and will produce strong signals after each 90° pulse. These tissues appear bright in the image.

The time between pulses is called the repetition time (TR). When the repetition time is very long, e.g., 4,000 msec, essentially all the body tissues have relaxed completely between pulses, so differences in T1 relaxation do not influence the signals generated. In other words, the final image contains no T1 information. If the repetition time is relatively short, e.g., 500 msec, some of the tissues do not have time to fully relax between pulses and produce weaker signals than if a long repetition time were used. These tissues are then said to be partially saturated. A pulse sequence that is rapidly repeated is often called a partial saturation sequence. The shorter the repetition time, the more saturated the tissues will be, and the relative signal differences between tissues will depend more and more on differences in T1, the rate of longitudinal relaxation.

Images whose content is dependent primarily on T1 properties can be made using another pulse sequence called inversion recovery (IR). In this sequence, two RF pulses are delivered in tandem. The first RF pulse is twice as long (or strong) as a 90° pulse, so it actually inverts M or flips it by 180°. As the protons relax back toward their original alignment, the inverted magnetization first recedes along the Z axis shrinking in net magnitude; then it increases again as the magnetization reaccumulates in the direction of B_0 (Fig. 10).

The rate at which this longitudinal relaxation occurs is described by T1, but no signal is generated as long as the magnetization is aligned with the Z axis. If another pulse of 90° duration is applied at some point in the relaxation process, then M will be flipped into the transverse plane, and a signal will be generated (Fig. 11). The amplitude of this signal depends on the magnitude of M when it

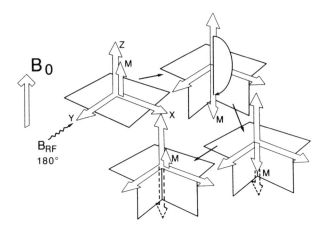

FIG. 10. Inversion recovery.

was flipped into the transverse plane. In other words, the 90° pulse enables us to measure M at some point in the longitudinal relaxation process. Different tissues have different rates of relaxation and will produce signals of differing strength and thus will appear with differing degrees of brightness in the image (Figs. 12 and 13). The IR sequence therefore produces an image based on relative differences in T1, so it is said to be T1-weighted.

The interpulse delay time between the 180° pulse and the following 90° pulse is called the inversion time (TI). TIs on the order of 400 to 700 msec are commonly used in clinical imaging. The time between the beginning of one tandem 180°-TI-90° pulse sequence and the beginning of the next one is the repetition time. A typical TR would be about 1,500 msec or longer for an IR 400 sequence (Fig. 14).

The spin–echo sequence is used to create an image dependent mainly on T2. Again, a tandem pulse sequence is employed, but this time a 90° pulse is followed by a 180° pulse. After the 90° pulse, the protons begin to dephase, some precessing slightly faster than others. Dephasing is partly due to spin–spin interactions and

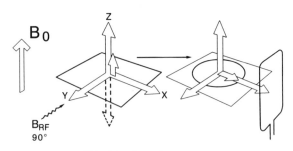

FIG. 11. Inversion recovery.

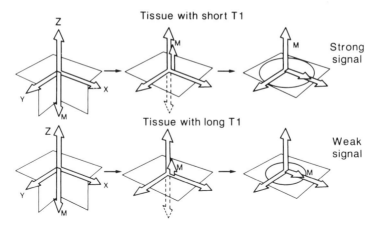

FIG. 12. Inversion recovery.

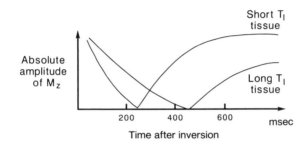

FIG. 13. Inversion recovery.

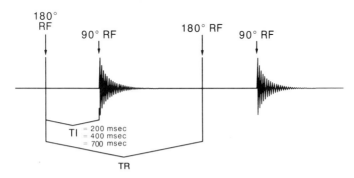

FIG. 14. Inversion recovery: T1 weighted; TR $\simeq$ 1,000–4,000 msec repetition time.

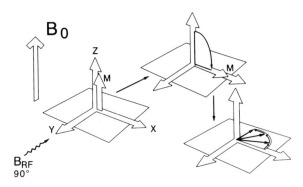

FIG. 15. Spin–echo.

partly due to inhomogeneities in the applied magnetic field (Fig. 15). After a certain interpulse delay time, the 180° pulse is applied. This flips the protons by 180° and essentially reverses their relative phase positions in the transverse plane. Now the faster precessing protons are behind the slower ones. As the faster ones catch up, the composite magnetization in the transverse plane builds to a peak again. It is this peak signal that we listen to or sample to create the image (Fig. 16).

The 180° pulse is a rephasing pulse that is used to reverse the effects of field inhomogeneity. Since true spin–spin interactions cannot be reversed by the rephasing pulse, the amplitude of the rephased signal is a reflection of the amount of true transverse relaxation that has occurred between the time of the 90° pulse and the peak echo signal. Different tissues have different rates of T2 relaxation, so their rephased signals differ in amplitude. Tissues with a long T2 relaxation time demonstrate little inherent dephasing and produce strong echoes. Tissues with short T2 relaxation times dephase more completely, so their rephased signals are smaller in amplitude, and these tissues appear relatively dark in the image.

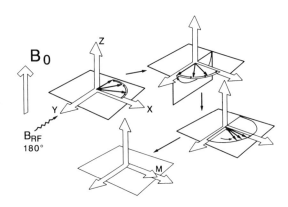

FIG. 16. Spin–echo.

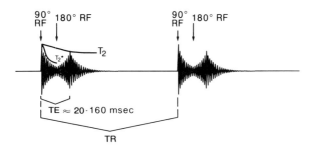

FIG. 17. Spin–echo: T2 or T1 weighted; TR $\simeq$ 150–4,000 msec repetition time.

Note that the time from the 90° pulse to the peak echo is called the echo time (TE). Note also that the TE is determined by the length of the interpulse delay time. Various interpulse delay times can be chosen for clinical imaging, resulting in echo times ranging typically from 20 to 160 msec (Fig. 17). Using longer interpulse delay times, and thus longer TE, results in accentuation of the contrast between tissues with different T2 relaxation rates, since there is more time for these differences in relaxation to express themselves before the echo is generated (Fig. 18). In other words, longer TE produces more T2 dependence in the image. Unfortunately, using longer TE also results in weaker echoes because of the inherent dephasing over time. The signal-to-noise ratio decreases, so the image looks more noisy, and anatomic definition is adversely affected.

Spin–echo sequences that have a short TE are relatively less T2-weighted than those with long TEs. Decreasing T2 dependence in the image has the effect of relatively increasing T1 dependence. Shortening the TR also introduces more T1 dependence in the image because of the saturation effect as described above. Thus, a spin–echo technique with a very short TE and a very short TR is referred to as a partial saturation sequence, and it produces an image that is T1-weighted. Therefore, spin–echo sequences can be either T1- or T2-weighted, depending on the pulse timing used.

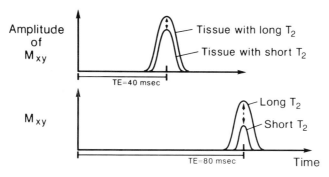

FIG. 18. Spin–echo.

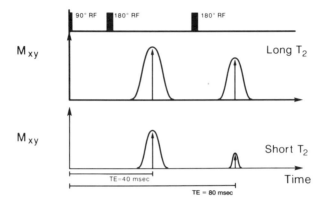

FIG. 19. Multiple spin–echo.

Another variation of the spin–echo sequence is called the Carr–Purcell–Mei-boom–Gill (CPMG) method of producing multiple spin–echoes. In this sequence, a 90° RF pulse is then followed by two or more 180° rephasing pulses. This produces two or more spin–echoes from which two or more images of the same slice are formed with progressively increasing T2 dependence (Fig. 19).

Let us now discuss how the magnetic fields are created and how spatial localization and RF stimulation are accomplished for cross-sectional imaging. The two most common magnetic devices employed in clinical imaging are the resistive and the superconducting types of magnets. Both are essentially large electromagnets, since they utilize circular flowing electric current to produce a strong field in the center of the magnet. Electric current flowing in a wire produces a surrounding magnetic field. A stronger field can be produced by current flowing in multiple loops of wire wound into a coil. Several coils can be lined up to produce a summated field if the current flowing around the coils is in the same direction (Figs. 20 and 21).

The resistive magnet typically consists of four large coils, each made of aluminum sheets wrapped many times around a simple supporting structure. Current flowing in the aluminum produces the magnetic field. There is resistance in the aluminum to the flow of electric current, hence the name resistive magnet.

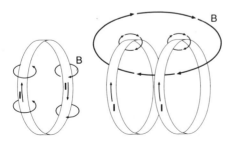

FIG. 20. Magnetic field.

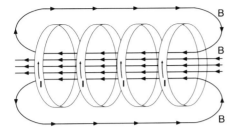

FIG. 21. Magnetic field.

A resistive magnet consumes a considerable amount of electricity, which adds to operating costs, and it generates much heat, requiring air- and water-cooling systems to prevent overheating. However, a resistive magnet costs less to purchase than a superconducting system, and it weighs less and requires less shielding of the magnetic field. Conventional resistive magnets produce fields up to approximately 0.15 T.

Superconducting or cryogenic magnets have coils usually made of niobium–titanium wire embedded in a copper matrix. Liquid helium is used to cool the coils to near absolute zero. At this temperature, electric current flows without resistance, hence the name superconducting. Liquid nitrogen is used to surround and insulate the liquid helium from the ambient room temperature. Superconductors create fields for clinical imaging up to 1.5 T and are necessary to produce the very high fields required for spectroscopy. They also create more homogeneous magnetic fields than do resistive systems; this is an important factor in image quality. Operating costs of a superconductor result primarily from the consumption of liquid helium and nitrogen. Site considerations may be more complex with a superconducting system than a resistive system, since it weighs more and may require much steel shielding to decrease the field strength around the perimeter of the imaging area. Proper ventilation is needed to remove the gases that boil off during every day use or that might flood the room otherwise in the event of quenching of the superconducting magnet.

Rather than using an electromagnet, some MR imagers employ a large permanent magnet to create the main static field. These magnets are composed of blocks of permanently magnetized material and are assembled on site. Permanent fields up to 0.3 T are created without the operating costs of a resistive or superconducting system. These magnets are generally very heavy.

The main magnet of an MR imager produces the stationary field B_0. Inside the magnet are other coils: the RF coils, which allow stimulation of the hydrogen protons and reception of their signals, and the gradient coils, which are essential for spatial localization of these signals

It was stated earlier in the chapter that the Larmor frequency is directly related to the magnetic field strength. In other words, any change in the field strength produces a proportional change in the frequency of precession. This is the key principle that allows for spatial localization in MR imaging. The gradient coils

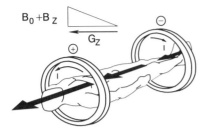

FIG. 22. Z-gradient coils.

FIG. 23. Z-gradient coils.

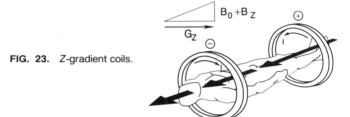

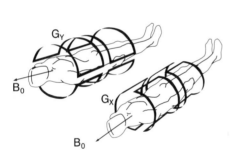

FIG. 24. X and Y gradient coils.

alter the main magnetic field B_0 so that different parts of the body experience a different field strength. Those protons in a stronger field will precess faster than those protons in a nearby weaker field. Therefore, resonant frequency will vary according to location.

A pair of circular coils near the ends of the magnet make up the Z-gradient coils. A gradient in the Z direction means that the strength of the magnetic field changes with reference to position along the Z axis. The direction of change is the direction of the gradient. This direction can be switched at will electronically by altering the current flow in the two gradient coils. Note that a gradient can be made to change directions, but the overall magnetic field is always oriented in the same direction (Figs. 22 and 23).

The X and Y gradient coils have a saddle shape. Coils above and below the patient create the Y gradient. A similar set on both sides of the patient creates the X gradient (Fig. 24).

For transaxial imaging, slice selection is accomplished by the application of the Z gradient during RF stimulation. Because of the gradient in the magnetic

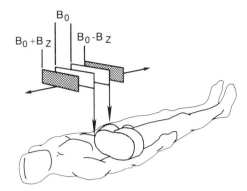

FIG. 25. Selective excitation technique.

field, each sectional plane of the body experiences a different magnetic field, and only one plane near the center of the area of interest will experience a field strength equal to B_0. If an RF pulse is then applied with a frequency exactly equal to the Larmor frequency appropriate for B_0 then only those protons in this one plane of tissue will be caused to resonate and thus produce an MR signal. This method of slice selection is referred to as the selective excitation technique (Fig. 25). Slice thickness depends on the steepness of the slope in the field gradient and the bandwidth or range of frequencies contained in the RF pulse. A narrower range of frequencies will excite a thinner slice of tissue. To image in the coronal plane, the X-gradient field is applied during RF stimulation to select the slice. For sagittal imaging, the Y gradient is used. Multiplanar imaging is of course one of the principal advantages of MR imaging:

> *Transaxial imaging*—slice selection, Z gradient; transverse localization, X, Y gradients.
> *Coronal imaging*—slice selection, Y gradient.
> *Sagittal imaging*—slice selection, X gradient.

After the slice has been selected during RF stimulation, spatial localization within the slice needs to be accomplished. A method of data acquisition commonly used to do this is called a two-dimensional Fourier transformation (2DFT). This involves using the two gradients not used in slice selection, e.g., the X and Y gradients in the case of transaxial imaging, to encode the proton signals with certain labels that will reveal their origin within the slice. These two gradients are applied in succession after RF stimulation. The first gradient will cause the proton signals to be slightly offset in phase in relation to each other, depending on their positions in space along the axis of this gradient. The signals are then said to be phase encoded. The second gradient, called the frequency encoding or read-out gradient, is applied when the precessing protons are emitting their signals. With this gradient applied, those protons on the side of the slice experiencing the strongest field will precess faster than those protons on the other side experiencing a weaker field, as dictated by the Larmor relationship. In other words, the protons will precess at different rates or with different frequencies

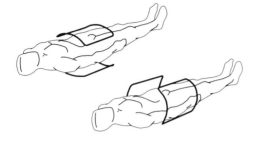

FIG. 26. Radiofrequency coils: transmitter–receiver.

FIG. 27. Radiofrequency field, B_1.

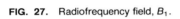

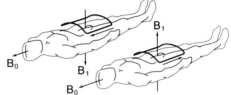

related to their positions along the axis of the frequency-encoding gradient in the field. So the RF receiver coils pick up multiple signals that have both phase and frequency labels that describe their location. Either 128 or 256 phase-encoding views of the slice are obtained each using a different slope in the gradient to label the proton signals with greater amounts of phase shift each time in order to localize them more precisely in space. A constant number of frequency dimensions, e.g., 256, are established by the frequency-encoding gradient for each view. The data from the different views are decoded using Fourier transformation (FT), and an image is formed. In others words, a checkerboard-type matrix is created, with the protons in each box giving signals that have a unique combination of phase and frequency labels that identify their location within the slice. The box is really a volume of tissue determined by the matrix size and the thickness of the slice selected. This volume element is called a voxel. The amplitude of the proton signals from this voxel are determined by the spin density and the relaxation characteristics of the tissue within the voxel. If the average amplitude is large, the voxel is assigned a bright or high-intensity value in the image. If the amplitude is small, it is assigned a low-intensity value. Voxel refers to the three-dimensional volume of tissue producing the signal. The result is visualized as a picture element, or pixel, in the two-dimensional image.

The RF coils are made of copper and have a saddle shape similar to the X and Y gradient coils (Fig. 26). Current flowing in the transmitter coil creates a magnetic field B_1 perpendicular to the larger static magnetic field B_0. The current in the transmitter coil and the resulting B_1 field switch direction with a frequency equal to the Larmor frequency (Fig. 27). In this way, energy is delivered to the tissue of interest at a frequency that matches the frequency of the precessing protons, and resonance occurs. Improved signals are obtained with receiver coils being located as close to the tissue of interest as possible, so a smaller set of receiver coils are used for imaging the head and extremities, compared to those used for the body trunk. In addition, separate movable surface coils have been developed that can be closely applied to the body for specific imaging of a smaller volume of interest close to the body surface, such as the orbit, spine, or peripheral joint.

GLOSSARY[1]

Acquisition time   Time needed to acquire the raw data from an MR procedure. Additional reconstruction time is needed to formulate the image before it can actually be viewed.

B_0 Symbol for the constant magnetic field, referring to units of magnetic induction or T.

B_1 Symbol for the RF magnetic induction field or the RF pulse.

Chemical shift   The change in the Larmor frequency of a given nucleus, e.g., hydrogen or phosphorus when bound in different sites within a molecule, due to the magnetic shielding effects of nearby orbiting electrons. The amount of shift increases with increasing field strength. It is usually specified in parts per million (ppm) of the resonance frequency relative to a standard.

Coil   Single or multiple loops of wire (or other electrical conductor, such as tubing) designed either to produce a magnetic field from electric current flowing through the wire, or to detect a changing magnetic field by voltage induced in the wire.

Eddy currents   Electric currents induced in a conductor by a changing magnetic field or by motion of the conductor through a magnetic field.

Excitation   Putting energy into the spin system.

Ferromagnetic   A substance such as iron that can be easily magnetized.

Flip angle   Amount of rotation of *M* produced by an RF pulse, with respect to the direction of the static magnetic field B_0.

Fourier transform (FT)   A mathematical procedure to separate out the frequency components of a signal from its amplitudes as a function of time or vice versa.

Free induction decay (FID)   A transient MR signal resulting when magnetization in the transverse plane is produced, e.g., by a 90° RF pulse. This decaying signal is the FID. The rate of decay is described by T2 star (T2*).

Frequency   The number of repetitions of a periodic process per unit time. For electromagnetic radiation, such as radiowaves, the old unit, cycles per second, has been replaced by hertz (Hz), under the preferred International System of Units (SI). One million hertz equals one megahertz (MHz).

G_x, G_y, G_z Conventional symbols for gradient magnetic fields. Used with subscripts to denote the spatial direction along which the field changes.

Gauss (G)   A unit of magnetic flux density. The earth's magnetic field is approximately

---

[1] This list has been selected and adapted from the more comprehensive and precise *Glossary of NMR Terms* (5).

one-half to one G, depending on location. The currently preferred (SI) unit is the tesla (T). One T equals 10,000 G or 10 kilogauss (kG).

Gradient   The amount and direction of the rate of change in space of some quantity such as magnetic field strength.

Gradient coils   Current carrying coils designed to produce a desired gradient magnetic field.

Gradient magnetic field   A magnetic field that changes in strength in a given certain direction.

Gyromagnetic ratio   The ratio of the magnetic moment to the angular momentum of a particle. This is a constant for a given nucleus.

Homogeneity   Uniformity. The homogeneity of the static magnetic field is an important criterion of the quality of the magnet.

Inhomogeneity   Degree of lack of homogeneity.

Interpulse time   Time between successive RF pulses within a pulse sequence.

Inversion   A nonequilibrium state in which M is oriented opposite to the magnetic field.

Inversion recovery (IR)   Pulse technique wherein the nuclear magnetization is inverted at a time on the order of T1 before the regular imaging pulse gradient sequences.

Inversion time (TI)   Time between the inverting 180° pulse and the subsequent 90° pulse to elicit MR signal in IR.

Larmor equation   States that the frequency of precession of the nuclear magnetic moment is proportional to the magnetic field.

Lattice   The magnetic and thermal environment with which nuclei exchange energy in longitudinal relaxation.

Longitudinal magnetization   See M_z.

Longitudinal relaxation   Return of longitudinal magnetization (M_z) to its equilibrium value after excitation; requires exchange of energy between the nuclear spins and the lattice.

M   Conventional symbol for macroscopic magnetization vector—net magnetic moment per unit volume of a sample in a given region, considered as the integrated effect of all the individual microscopic nuclear magnetic moments.

$M_{x,y}$ Transverse magnetization—component of M at right angles to the static magnetic field (B_0). Precession of the transverse magnetization at the Larmor frequency is responsible for the detectable MR signal. In the absence of externally applied RF energy, the transverse magnetization will decay to zero with a characteristic time constant of T2 or T2*.

M_z Longitudinal magnetization—Component of M along the static magnetic field. Following excitation by an RF pulse, M_z will approach its equilibrium value with a characteristic time constant T1.

Macroscopic magnetization vector   See *M*.

Magnetic dipole   North and south magnetic poles separated by a finite distance.

Magnetic field   The region surrounding a magnet (or current carrying conductor) is endowed with certain properties. One is that a small magnet in such a region experiences a torque that tends to align it in a given direction. Magnetic field is a vector quantity; the direction of the field is defined as the direction that the north pole of the small magnet points when in equilibrium. A magnetic field produces a magnetizing force on a body within it.

Magnetic moment   A measure of the net magnetic properties of an object or particle. A nucleus with an intrinsic spin will have an associated magnetic dipole moment, so that it will interact with a magnetic field (as if it were a tiny bar magnet).

Paramagnetic   A substance with a small but positive magnetic susceptibility (magnetizability). The addition of a small amount of paramagnetic substance may greatly reduce the relaxation times of water. Typical paramagnetic substances usually possess an unpaired electron and include atoms or ions of transition elements, rare earth elements, some metals, and some molecules including molecular oxygen and free radicals. Paramagnetic substances are sometimes used as contrast agents in MR imaging.

Partial saturation (PS)   Excitation technique applying repeated RF pulses in times on the order of or shorter than T1.

Phase   In a periodic function (such as rotational or sinusoidal motion), the position relative to a particular part of the cycle.

Pixel   Acronym for a picture element; the smallest discrete part of a digital image display.

Precession   Comparatively slow gyration of the axis of a spinning body so as to trace out a cone. A familiar example is the effect of gravity on the motion of a spinning top or gyroscope.

Quenching   Loss of superconductivity of the current carrying coil that may occur unexpectedly in a superconducting magnet. As the magnet becomes resistive, heat will be released, which can result in rapid evaporation of liquid helium.

Radiofrequency (RF)   Wave frequency intermediate between auditory and infrared.

Repeated FID   A form of MR imaging in which repeated 90° pulses are applied. Results in partial saturation if interpulse times are of the order of or less than T1.

Resistive magnet   A magnet whose magnetic field originates from current flowing through an ordinary (nonsuperconducting) conductor.

Resonance   A large amplitude vibration in a mechanical or electrical system caused by a relatively small periodic stimulus with a frequency at or close to a natural frequency of the system.

RF pulse   Brief burst of RF magnetic field delivered to object by RF transmitter.

Saturation   A nonequilibrium state in MR, in which equal numbers of spins are aligned against and with the magnetic field, so that there is no net magnetization.

Selective excitation   Controlling the frequency spectrum of an irradiating RF pulse while imposing a gradient magnetic field on spins, such that only a desired region will have a suitable resonant frequency to be excited.

Shim coils   Coils carrying a relatively small current that are used to provide auxiliary magnetic fields in order to compensate for inhomogeneities in the main magnetic field of an MR system.

Shimming   Correction of inhomogeneity of the magnetic field produced by the main magnet of an MR system due to imperfections in the magnet or to the presence of external ferromagnetic objects. May involve changing the configuration of the magnet or the addition of shim coils or small pieces of steel.

Signal-to-noise ratio (SNR or S/N)   Used to describe the relative contributions to a detected signal of the true signal and random superimposed signals (noise).

Spectrum   An array of the frequency components of the MR signal according to frequency. Nuclei with different resonant frequencies will show up as peaks at different corresponding frequencies in the spectrum, or lines.

Spin   The intrinsic angular momentum of an elementary particle, or system of particles such as a nucleus, that is also responsible for the magnetic moment; or, a particle or nucleus possessing such a spin.

Spin density (N)   The density of resonating spins in a given region.

Spin-echo   Reappearance of an MR signal after the FID has died away, as a result of the effective reversal of the dephasing of the spins (refocusing).

Spin–lattice relaxation time   See T1.

Spin–spin relaxation time   See T2.

Spin warp imaging   A form of FT imaging in which phase-encoding gradient pulses are applied for a constant duration but with varying amplitude.

Superconducting magnet   A magnet whose magnetic field originates from current flowing through a superconductor.

Superconductor   A substance whose electrical resistance essentially disappears at temperatures near absolute zero.

Surface coil   A simple flat RF receiver coil placed over a region of interest will have an effective selectivity for a volume approximately subtended by the coil circumference and one radius deep from the coil center.

T1 ("T-one")   Spin–lattice or longitudinal relaxation time; the characteristic time constant for spins to tend to align themselves with the external magnetic field. Starting from zero magnetization in the z direction, the z magnetization will grow to 63% of its final maximum value in a time T1.

T2 ("T-two")   Spin–spin or transverse relaxation time; the characteristic time constant for loss of phase coherence among spins oriented at an angle to the static magnetic field, due to interactions between the spins, with resulting loss of transverse magnetization and nuclear magnetic resonance signal. Starting from a nonzero value of the magnetization in the x,y plane, the x,y magnetization will decay so that it loses 63% of its initial value in a time T2.

T2* ("T-two-star")   The characteristic time constant for loss of phase coherence among spins oriented at an angle to the static magnetic field due to a combination of magnetic field inhomogeneities and spin–spin transverse relaxation with resultant more rapid loss in transverse magnetization and MR signal.

TE   Echo time. Time between middle of 90° pulse and middle of spin–echo production. For multiple echoes, use TE1, TE2, etc.

Tesla (T)   The preferred (SI) unit of magnetic flux density. One T is equal to 10,000 G, the older (CGS) unit.

TI   Inversion time. Time after middle of inverting RF pulse to middle of 90° pulse to detect amount of longitudinal magnetization.

TR   Repetition time. The period of time between the beginning of a pulse sequence and the beginning of the succeeding (essentially identical) pulse sequence.

Transverse magnetization   *See* $M_{x,y}$.

Transverse relaxation time   *See* T2.

Two-dimensional Fourier transform imaging (2DFT)   A form of sequential plane imaging using FT imaging.

Tuning   Process of adjusting the resonant frequency, e.g., of the RF circuit, to a desired value, e.g., the Larmor frequency.

Vector   A quantity having both magnitude and direction, frequently represented by an arrow whose length is proportional to the magnitude and with an arrowhead at one end to indicate the direction.

Voxel   Volume element; the element of three-dimensional space corresponding to a pixel, for a given slice thickness.

BIBLIOGRAPHY

Andrew, E. R., and Worthington, B. S. (1981): Nuclear magnetic resonance imaging. In: *Radiology of the Skull and Brain,* edited by T. H. Newton and D. G. Potts, Chapter 132, pp. 4389–4405. C. V. Mosby, St. Louis.

Bydder, G. M., and Steiner, R. E. (1982): NMR imaging of the brain. *Neuroradiology,* 23:231–240.

Crooks, L., et al. (1982): Nuclear magnetic resonance whole-body images operating at 3.5 KGauss. *Radiology,* 143:169–174.

Fullerton, G. D. (1982): Basic concepts for nuclear magnetic resonance imaging. *Magnetic Resonance Imaging,* 1:39–55.

Glossary of NMR Terms (1983): American College of Radiology, Chicago. [Booklet.]

Gore, J. C., et al. (1981): Medical nuclear magnetic resonance imaging: 1. Physical principles. *Invest. Radiol.,* 16:269–274.

McCullough, E. C., and Baker, H. L., Jr. (1982): Nuclear magnetic resonance imaging. *Radiol. Clin. North. Am.,* 20:3–7.

Pykett, I. L., et al. (1982): Principles of nuclear magnetic resonance imaging. *Radiology,* 143:157–168.

Pykett, I. L. (1982): NMR imaging in medicine. *Sci. Am.,* 246:78–88.

Interpretation of Magnetic Resonance Images

Richard L. Ehman

Mayo Medical School, and Department of Diagnostic Radiology, Mayo Clinic, Rochester, Minnesota 55905

Magnetic resonance (MR) images are based on an entirely different set of physical principles than X-ray-based or other familiar medical imaging techniques. This presents both a problem and an opportunity to physicians who must interpret these images. It is a problem because we have no background of intuitive knowledge to draw from in order to understand the pattern of black, white, and grey that is present in the images. It is an opportunity because, as MR imaging is based on a unique set of physical principles, it is inevitable that some tissue interfaces will be displayed with higher clarity than with other imaging modalities. The challenge for any physician who would like to employ this powerful technique is therefore to gain a working understanding of the MR properties of tissue and how they are portrayed in the images.

The purpose of this chapter is to describe the properties of tissue that are important in MR imaging of the musculoskeletal system. The dependence of these physical properties on tissue type and pathology is still poorly understood, but some of the general principles are useful in clinical practice. We will outline methods for tailoring MR examinations to make appropriate use of this information for common clinical problems. Approaches for interpreting image contrast will be presented. The physical mechanisms that govern the appearance of flowing blood will also be covered.

TISSUE CHARACTERIZATION

The process of extracting information about tissue type and pathology by MR techniques has been called tissue characterization. This is usually regarded as a method involving quantitative measurement of relaxation times. Many studies of tissue characterization by *in vivo* measurement of relaxation times have appeared in the literature (13,30,33,36,40,49). These have generally not demon-

23

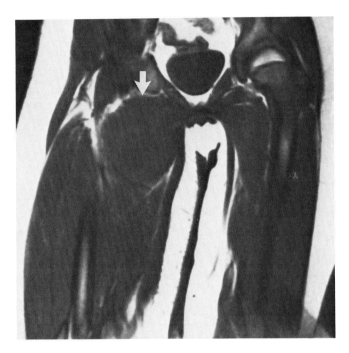

FIG. 1. Malignant soft tissue tumor (*arrow*) which is differentiated from muscle on the basis of its mass effect and homogeneity rather than a contrast difference.

strated a strong clinical role for tissue characterization, although it is fair to say that the hypothesis that accurate measurement of tissue relaxation times may be clinically useful has not yet been adequately tested.

It should be remembered at this point that tissue characterization is not something that is limited to MR. It is performed in every branch of diagnostic imaging. Consider the case of a solitary pulmonary nodule that is observed in a chest radiograph. If a certain pattern of calcification is identified within the nodule it can be judged benign. Other examples include assessing whether a mass is cystic or solid with ultrasonography and determining the presence or absence of fat within a renal mass with computed tomography (CT). These processes are mostly qualitative, based on an understanding of the grey scale of the particular imaging modality. Some can be quantitative, as with CT. In any case, all of these are examples of clinically useful tissue characterization. We believe that it is this type of tissue characterization, based on knowledge and manipulation of tissue contrast that is most important in clinical MR imaging.

Given the expanded definition for tissue characterization described above, what are the properties that are important in clinical imaging? A key word in this question is "imaging." Some of the tissue properties that are important in this context are unique to the imaging process. This includes anatomic detail which can demonstrate a lesion solely by its effect on morphology (Fig. 1). Another similar property is tissue texture: mass lesions in muscle are often characterized by their homogeneous texture, compared to the reticulated texture of normal muscle (Fig. 1). As we shall see, even some of the classic tissue characterization parameters have special meanings in the imaging context.

MR images basically reflect the distribution of mobile hydrogen nuclei. The brightness of each image pixel depends, among other things, on the density of mobile protons in the corresponding volume element and on the way that these protons respond to the externally superimposed static and fluctuating magnetic fields described in the previous chapter (J. Nixon, *this volume*). This response depends on the chemical and biophysical environment of the protons and is described concisely by the relaxation times T1 and T2.

The spin–lattice relaxation time, T1, is an exponential time constant which describes the gradual increase in magnetization that takes place when a substance is placed in a strong magnetic field (Fig. 2). It predicts the time that it will take for nearly two-thirds (actually approximately 63%) of the longitudinal magnetization to be restored after it has been tipped 90° by a radiofrequency (RF) pulse. The spin–lattice relaxation time of water protons in tissue depends in a complex fashion on rotational, vibrational, and translational motions and on the way that these are modified by proximity to macromolecules.

The spin–spin relaxation time, T2, is a time constant that describes the rate of exponential decay of transverse magnetization that would occur if the field was perfectly homogeneous (Fig. 3). Thus, with the spin–echo technique, if an echo is created at a time (TE) equal to the TR relaxation time, the transverse magnetization will have decayed away by a factor of approximately 2/3 (actually, 63%) from what was present immediately after the 90° pulse. The transverse magnetization is the component that creates a signal in MR imaging. Like T1, the spin–spin relaxation time depends on the natural motions of molecules. It is also affected by other processes which will be described later in this chapter.

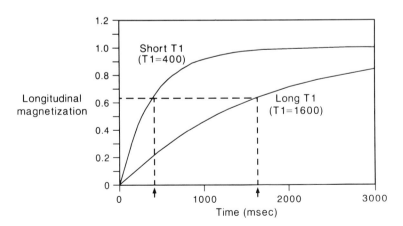

FIG. 2. The T1 relaxation time describes the regrowth of longitudinal magnetization after it is reduced to zero by a 90° RF pulse.

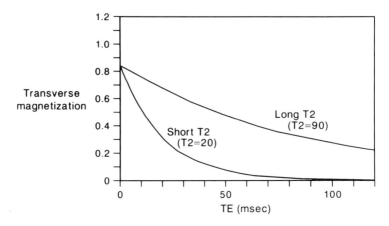

Transverse magnetization

TE (msec)

FIG. 3.   The T2 relaxation time describes the exponential decay of magnetization in the transverse plane after it is placed there by a 90° RF pulse.

Accurate *in vivo* measurement of relaxation times is difficult with most MR imagers. These difficulties relate to the necessity of irradiating a large but well-defined volume with RF energy and performing the steps required to create an image. Slice-selective 90 and 180° RF pulses, for instance, tend to be inaccurate near the boundaries of the section (28). The signal obtained from tissue which is irradiated with inaccurate RF pulses will not be the same as what would be obtained with ideal pulses. Relaxation times calculated from such measurements will be correspondingly incorrect. Other problems include the effects of applied field gradients, motion, and the small number of data points that are typically acquired.

In spite of these problems, properly performed *in vivo* relaxation time measurements are surprisingly reproducible with the same imager when they are performed on tissues that are stationary (29,30). On the other hand, physiological motion can produce large random and systematic errors in relaxation times calculated from image data (15,16). Relaxation times obtained with one type of MR imager are usually not directly comparable to data obtained for the same tissue with another imager. This is because of the imager-specific systematic errors described above and the fact that relaxation times are field strength dependent. The T1 of muscle tissue, for instance, is nearly twice as long at 1.5 T as it is at 0.15 T (4,26).

Given these problems, it is not surprising that clinical applications requiring quantitative measurement of tissue relaxation times have been slow to emerge. In spite of this, it is essential to understand the relative relaxation time relationships of tissues and pathological processes because this is the key to understanding the highly variable grey scale of MR imaging.

Spin density (mobile proton density; hydrogen density) is another important property that determines the appearance of tissue in MR images. Few *in vivo* measurements of tissue spin density have been reported. This is probably because absolute measurements are difficult to perform with imagers. The derived spin densities are relative values that can only be compared within the same image. Nevertheless, spin density differences are an important source of image contrast in some tissues. There are large differences between the spin density of adipose tissue and muscle, for instance (14).

Many other physical properties can potentially be measured or monitored by MR techniques in order to noninvasively characterize tissue. These include measuring the diffusion rate of water protons (46,47) and differentiating between groups of protons on the basis of the characteristic chemical shift in their resonant frequency (11,18,27,32,38,48).

SIGNIFICANCE OF TISSUE RELAXATION TIMES

A detailed discussion of the physical mechanisms that determine relaxation time in biological systems is beyond the scope of this chapter. Indeed, these processes are as yet relatively poorly understood. Nevertheless, some of the concepts in the current view of this area are useful for understanding the appearance of normal and pathological tissue in clinical images.

Relaxation times are used to describe the time course of the bulk magnetization of resonating protons following the application of perturbing RF pulses. The bulk magnetization is a vector quantity (i.e., having a magnitude and direction) which is the sum of the minute magnetic contributions of each of the resonating protons in tissue. The magnetic behavior of individual protons is quantum mechanical in nature, but the process of summing huge numbers of protons results in a bulk magnetization vector (M) which can assume a continuous range of magnitudes and orientations.

As already noted, the spin–lattice relaxation time (T1) describes the restoration of the longitudinal component of magnetization after it has been tipped by an RF pulse. In order for this to happen, some of the protons that have been boosted into a higher energy level by the RF pulse must give up energy to the surrounding environment (sometimes called the lattice). This corresponds to reorienting individual proton magnetic moments from a direction that is roughly opposite to that of the main field to one that is, on average, in the same direction.

This process depends on interaction between the excited protons and neighboring nuclei in the lattice (17). The protons are subjected to a rapidly varying perturbation by the magnetic fields of adjacent nuclei. The frequency with which they vary is determined by the tumbling and translational motions of the protons and their neighbors. The perturbing motions are most effective for stimulating spin–lattice relaxation when they fluctuate at the Larmor frequency of the system.

The characteristic length of time during which the magnetic field of a proton interacts with that of an adjacent nucleus with a magnetic moment is called the correlation time, τ (17). Essentially, this quantity is proportional to the period (i.e., inversely proportional to the frequency) of the cyclic field fluctuations caused by motion. Each mode of molecular motion has a characteristic correlation time. For tumbling motion, the correlation time is proportional to the period of rotation (Fig. 4). For translational motion, the correlation time can be regarded as proportional to the average time between the Brownian jumps. The combined correlation time is the parallel sum of the individual τ associated with each of the perturbing motions:

$$\frac{1}{\tau_c} = \frac{1}{\tau_r} + \frac{1}{\tau_d} \tag{1}$$

where τ_c is the net correlation time, τ_r the rotational correlation time, τ_d the correlation time associated with translational motion.

As shown in Fig. 5, the spin–lattice relaxation time decreases to a minimum as correlation time is lengthened and then increases again. The position of the minimum of this curve is dependent on the Larmour frequency and thus the strength of the B_0 field (3). Free water has a short correlation time of about 10^{-12} sec, and thus it has a long spin–lattice relaxation time.

The spin–spin or T2 relaxation time of protons is also dependent on correlation times. It is also strongly affected by slowly varying and static magnetic fields at the molecular level (17). Such fields form gradients which cause moving protons to precess at rates which have a small random variation with time. Thus they do not stay in phase with each other for as long as they would without the static field gradients and this is reflected as a reduction in the T2 relaxation time (see J. Nixon, *this volume*). Figure 5 shows that, in contrast to the T1 relaxation time, T2 continues to shorten as correlation times become longer and longer. Thus, the proton T1 and T2 relaxation times of solids that have very slow molecular motion and longer correlation times will be long and short, respectively.

Although pure water has long T1 and T2 relaxation times of over 2 sec, much shorter relaxation times are typically observed in tissue. This is a result of the hydrophilic properties of many macromolecules. These molecules, which include proteins and polynucleic acids, have electric dipole and ionic sites, which allow hydrogen bonding with water molecules in solution (Fig. 6) (10,21,23). The water in this hydration layer is less mobile than free water and thus the correlation time is longer (τ_c on the order of 10^{-9} sec). As a result, the T1 and T2 of bound water is much shorter than that of free water.

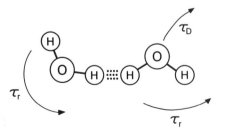

FIG. 4. As water molecules tumble and randomly jump in Brownian motion, the dipole moments of protons interact with a characteristic period which is called the correlation time.

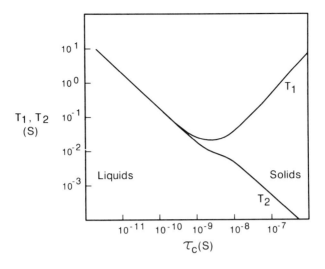

FIG. 5.   Relationship between correlation time and the T1 and T2 relaxation times.

The residence time of individual water molecules in the hydration layer of macromolecules is transient. Thus, individual water protons may alternately experience conditions which are favorable and unfavorable for relaxation as they exchange back and forth between bound and free states, respectively. Under these fast exchange conditions, the observed relaxation time of water protons will be an average of the relaxation times in the bound and free states, weighted by the fraction in each state (10):

$$\frac{1}{T1_o} = \frac{1 - F_b}{T1_f} + \frac{F_b}{T1_b} \qquad [2]$$

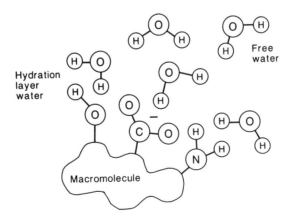

FIG. 6.   Two-state model for organization of water in cytoplasm.

where $T1_o$ is the observed $T1$, $T1_f$ and $T1_b$ are the relaxation times in the free and bound states, respectively, and F_b is the fraction of bound protons. The equation for T2 is similar. More complex models have been created to explain tissue relaxation behavior (4), but this simple, two-state, fast exchange model is very helpful for understanding clinical images. The T1 relaxation time of free water is approximately 2,500 msec, while that of hydration water is less than 100 msec. The model predicts that relaxation times of tissues with higher bound water fractions will be shorter than tissues that have a larger percentage of free water.

Tissue water proton relaxation times depend on many other factors. Field strength is one of the most important of these (4,9,20,26). The trough of the T1 relaxation time curve in Fig. 5 moves upward and to the left as field strength increases (3). This means that the relaxation times of protons with correlation times in this range (bound water protons, for instance) will be longer at higher field strengths. Thus, the T1 relaxation time of most tissues increases with field strength because of the influence on the bound water component. In contrast, the T2 relaxation times of most tissues are relatively independent of field strength, except for a clinically important situation described below.

Paramagnetic agents can strongly affect tissue relaxation times when they are present (7). These are substances with very strong magnetic moments which can enhance the relaxation of neighboring protons by perturbing them in a manner analogous to the way that proton fields interact with other protons. Many of these agents are paramagnetic by virtue of the presence of an unpaired orbital electron. The magnetic dipole moment generated by the unopposed electron is approximately 700 times stronger than the magnetic moment of a proton. The proton relaxation enhancement effect of these molecules is correspondingly intense.

When a sufficient amount of paramagnetic agent is added to an aqueous solution, the T1 and T2 relaxation times are shortened. The effect can be represented by the following equations:

$$\frac{1}{T1_o} = \frac{1}{T1_d} + \frac{1}{T1_p} \qquad [3]$$

$$\frac{1}{T2_o} = \frac{1}{T2_d} + \frac{1}{T2_p} \qquad [4]$$

where $T1_o$ and $T2_o$ are the new observed relaxation times, $T1_d$ and $T2_d$ are the (diamagnetic) relaxation times of the solution or tissue without the paramagnetic agent, and $T1_p$ and $T2_p$ represent the extra relaxation process provided by the addition of the paramagnetic material. These latter quantities depend on the concentration of paramagnetic material:

$$\frac{1}{T1_p} = K1 \times \text{concentration of paramagnetic material} \qquad [5]$$

$$\frac{1}{T2_p} = K2 \times \text{concentration of paramagnetic material} \qquad [6]$$

where K1 and K2 are constants that depend on the type of paramagnetic agent and on the characteristics of the tissue or solution.

Paramagnetic material may be endogenous in origin or it may be exogenously administered as a contrast agent for MR imaging. Endogenous paramagnetic materials are not believed to be present in sufficient concentration to significantly affect the relaxation behavior of most normal human tissues, but they do have a substantial effect in some pathological states such as transfusional hemosiderosis (8).

RELAXATION TIMES OF MUSCULOSKELETAL TISSUES

Tables of quantitative *in vivo* relaxation time measurements (4) are of limited clinical usefulness because they are dependent on field strength and technical details of the imager and measurement method. Nevertheless, a general understanding of the relative relaxation characteristics of normal and pathological tissues is absolutely essential for competent interpretation of clinical MR imagery. This task is relatively easy for the musculoskeletal system because the number of different tissues is small.

At the field strengths which are commonly used for proton imaging (0.15 to 1.5 T), the T1 relaxation times of most soft tissues range from 250 to 1,200 msec. The range of T2 values for most soft tissues is between approximately 25 and 120 msec. Fluids and fibrous tissue depart from this range. The relative relaxation times of musculoskeletal tissues are summarized in Table 1.

These relationships can be summarized in a relaxation time map (Fig. 7). This figure shows that most musculoskeletal soft tissues fall into three distinct classes. Adipose tissue is characterized by its short T1 relaxation time, short in comparison to most other tissues, which dominates its appearance with most common MR imaging techniques. Healthy skeletal muscle has a short T2 relaxation time that is characteristic. Most other soft tissues, including tumors, have T1 relaxation times that are longer than that of adipose tissue and T2 relaxation times that

TABLE 1. *Relative relaxation times of musculoskeletal tissues*

Tissue	T1	T2
Muscle	Medium	Short
Adipose tissue	Short	Medium
Nerve	Medium	Medium
Other soft tissue	Medium–long	Medium–long
Tendon, bone	—	Very short

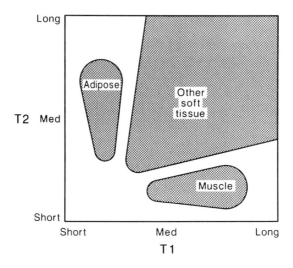

FIG. 7 Relaxation time map for musculoskeletal tissues.

are longer than that of muscle. The mobile proton density of bone, tendon, and dense fibrous tissue is low so that these tissues have low intensity in most MR images. These relationships form the basis for understanding and manipulating contrast in clinical MR of the musculoskeletal system.

EFFECT OF PATHOLOGY ON TISSUE RELAXATION TIMES

The relaxation times of many musculoskeletal tissues change in rather distinctive ways when they are affected by specific pathological processes. The significance and basic biophysical mechanisms for these changes are relatively poorly understood, and few clinical applications have been demonstrated for their quantitative measurement. However, they do cause diagnostically useful changes in the intensity and contrast of tissues in MR images. The general trend of the relaxation time changes for some important musculoskeletal disease processes is summarized in Table 2.

TABLE 2. *General trend of relaxation time changes for
some musculoskeletal disease processes*

Disease process	T1	T2
Inflammation	Increased	Increased
Neoplasia	Increased	Increased
Fibrosis	—	Decreased
Fatty infiltration	Decreased	—
Interstitial hemorrhage	Increased	Increased

Inflammation

Inflammatory processes are generally characterized by prolongation of T1 and T2 relaxation times (25). The presence of edema seems to be the most likely mechanism to explain these changes. Accumulation of extracellular and possibly intracellular water causes an increase in the total water content of tissue. The previously described two-state, fast exchange model is helpful for understanding how even a small change in water content can result in a large alteration in relaxation times. As water protons freely diffuse between the intracellular and extracellular spaces and the number of macromolecular binding sites is relatively fixed, the increased water content represents an increase in the fraction of free water

Figure 8 shows a simulation of observed tissue T1 values for various free water fractions, based on equation (2). The relaxation times $T1_f$ and $T1_b$ were assigned values of 2,500 and 50 msec, respectively. Relaxation time rapidly increases as the fraction of free water increases above 85%. Note, for instance that a 1% increase in free water from 91 to 92% causes a 10% increase in relaxation time.

Neoplasms

With certain exceptions, most solid neoplasms are characterized by relaxation times that are prolonged relative to their host tissues. Many studies of this phenomenon have appeared in the literature (2). Some studies have demonstrated increases in tissue water content that correlate with the degree of relaxation time prolongation, whereas others have not (10). The changes probably reflect an alteration in the ratio of free to bound water in tumor tissue, possibly related to changes in the way that water is ordered within and adjacent to the hydration layer of macromolecules.

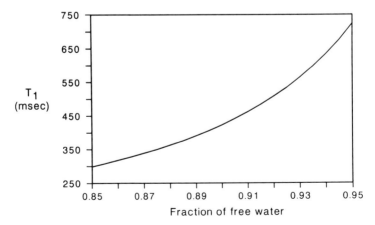

FIG. 8. Relationship between spin–lattice relaxation time and fraction of unbound or free water, using a fast exchange, two-state model for tissue relaxation times.

Although the elevation of T1 and T2 relaxation times in neoplastic tissue is often less than that resulting from inflammation, there is considerable overlap, and distinction between these processes must usually be made on the basis of morphology and the clinical setting.

Fibrosis

As noted above, the mobile spin density of predominantly fibrous tissue is low, thus providing little MR signal. Diffuse fibrosis of parenchymal tissues may be difficult to detect until it is well advanced and a substantial amount of the tissue has been replaced. The T2 relaxation time of fibrotic tissue is often reduced.

Fatty Infiltration

Fatty infiltration of muscles and other musculoskeletal tissues causes a shortening of *in vivo* T1 relaxation times because of the very short T1 of fat. A distinguishing feature between this and most other spin–lattice relaxation time changes related to disease is that the relaxation curves are not uniexponential (19). This is because there is little exchange between the protons in fat and those in the host tissue. The relaxation is therefore biexponential, with a fast component due to fat protons and a slower component due to water protons in the host tissue. Most *in vivo* methods for measuring T1 are incapable of resolving the biexponential nature of the recovery curve and simply report that the relaxation time is short.

Hematoma

Interstitial hemorrhage in muscle and other tissues usually causes prolongation of both T1 and T2 relaxation times, probably due to the presence of inflammation and edema (12,41).

The relaxation time characteristics of hematomas (confluent collections of extravasated blood) are much more variable. They are strongly influenced by formation of paramagnetic substances (5,22,41). Oxygenated hemoglobin contains iron in a low-spin ferrous state which is not paramagnetic. Thus, the proton relaxation times of stationary oxygenated blood are mainly determined by the concentration of protein (albumin and hemoglobin), which determines the fraction of water protons that are in the bound, fast-relaxing state. The T1 and T2 relaxation times of fresh oxygenated blood are medium or long in comparison to most solid tissue. Deoxygenation of hemoglobin has little effect on the relaxation time of hematomas at imager fields of less than 1.0 T. Deoxyhemoglobin contains iron in a high-spin ferrous state which is paramagnetic, but the area of the unpaired electron is relatively inaccessable to water protons because of the conformation of the molecule. Thus, the net relaxation of water protons is not enhanced, because they are unable to interact with the paramagnetic center.

As time passes, oxidative denaturation of deoxyhemoglobin causes formation of methemoglobin (5), which contains iron in a ferric form and is strongly paramagnetic. Water molecules have relatively free access to the paramagnetic site and thus the relaxation times are shortened. The T1 relaxation time of the hematoma is typically reduced more than T2 by the presence of methemoglobin. This can be understood by noting that the T2 of acute hematoma is short compared to its T1 relaxation time even though it is long in comparison to solid tissue. Even if $T1_p$ and $T2_p$ are relatively long, corresponding to a low concentration of methemoglobin, equations (3) and (4) show that $T1_o$ will be affected more than $T2_o$. For instance, if the $T1_d$ and $T2_d$ values of an acute hematoma are 600 and 150 msec, respectively, and after a period of time a small amount of methemoglobin is formed to yield paramagnetic contributions ($T1_p$ and $T2_p$) on the order of 1,000 msec, then the observed $T1_o$ and $T2_o$ values of the hematoma will be 375 and 130 msec, respectively. In a T1-weighted image (see next section) this would result in a substantial increase in intensity.

At higher field strengths (>1.0 T) an additional physical process begins to affect the relaxation times of hematogenous material. Empirical observations have shown that the T2 of hematomas can be extremely short at high field (1.5 T), whereas it is long in comparison to soft tissue at low and medium field strengths (22). The explanation of these observations relates to the fact that although deoxyhemoglobin is not an effective proton relaxation enhancer, it does cause the magnetic susceptibility of the erythrocyte cytoplasm to differ significantly from that of plasma. When a substance is placed in a magnetic field, the strength of the local magnetization typically differs from the external field strength by a proportionality factor called the bulk magnetic susceptibility.

The difference in magnetic susceptibility between plasma and cytoplasm results in a small difference in the field strength between the interior and exterior of erythrocytes. This gradient across the cell membranes is only 1 or 2 ten-thousandths of 1% (1 to 2 ppm) of the main magnetic field, but that is enough to shorten the T2 relaxation at high field (42). The mechanism is due to diffusion

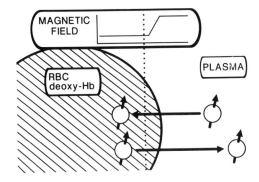

FIG. 9. Water protons diffusing through the cell membranes of erythrocytes containing deoxyhemoglobin (RBC deoxy-Hb) experience a tiny shift in their resonant frequency due to the presence of a field gradient. This causes selective reduction of T2 relaxation time at high field strengths.

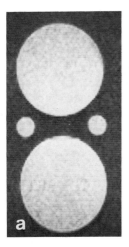 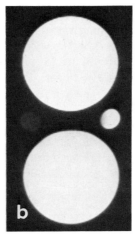

FIG. 10. Left: Low field T2-weighted image of two vials (small-diameter disks) containing blood. The image demonstrates no intensity difference between lysed blood in the tube on the right of the figure and intact cells in the tube on the left. The two large disks are reference standards. **Right:** High field T2-weighted image of same vials demonstrates striking reduction in the intensity of the nonlysed blood.

of water protons through the field gradients at the erythrocyte membrane (Fig. 9). Protons moving in such a fashion accumulate phase differences that would not have been present if the field gradients were absent, resulting in more rapid decay of the transverse magnetization. The phase errors are proportional to the square of the gradient. As the gradient is proportional to the field strength, this effect is much more pronounced at high field strength.

It is interesting to note that this T2 relaxation enhancement effect is operative only when erythrocyte membranes are intact. On lysis, the deoxyhemoglobin is distributed uniformly and the local field gradients abolished. Figure 10 shows a simple experiment in which two samples of diluted deoxygenated blood were imaged at 0.15 and 1.5 T. The sample on the right in the images was osmotically lysed. Note that both samples have identical intensity in a T2-weighted image (see next section) at 0.15 T, whereas the tube containing intact cells was dramatically reduced in intensity in a similar image at 1.5 T. The measured T2 relaxation times of both tubes at 0.15 T and the lysed tube at 1.5 T were greater than 150 msec. The T2 of the intact cells at 1.5 T was less than 45 msec.

Evidence indicates that a similar field-dependent T2 proton relaxation effect can also occur at the periphery of old hemorrhagic lesions due to susceptibility gradients in the vicinity of hemosiderin-laden macrophages (22).

In summary, the relaxation times of hematomas are affected by many factors, including protein concentration, formation of paramagnetic methemoglobin, and T2 proton relaxation enhancement by local heterogeneity in magnetic susceptibility at high field strength.

INFLUENCE OF RELAXATION TIMES AND PULSE SEQUENCE PARAMETERS ON CONTRAST

The appearance of tissue in clinical MR images depends on tissue properties and on the parameters of the pulse sequence. As already noted, the most important tissue properties in this context are the relaxation times T1 and T2 and the spin density N. The most important pulse sequence parameters are the pulse repetition time (TR) and the echo delay time (TE) for the spin–echo sequence. The inversion recovery (IR) sequence has an additional important parameter: inversion time (TI). In the discussion that follows, we will concentrate on the spin–echo technique as this is the most frequently used technique in current clinical MR imaging.

The importance of understanding the influence of these tissue properties and pulse sequence parameters on the contrast between tissues cannot be overstated. It provides a basis for characterizing tissue in clinical images. It also provides guidance for selecting appropriate MR imaging techniques from the huge number of possible parameter combinations so that the examination can be tailored to individual diagnostic problems.

Typical MR images are displayed in such a way that the brightness of each pixel is dependent on the MR signal that is obtained from each corresponding voxel (volume element) within the patient (Fig. 11). The precessing magnetization vector (M) in each volume element has a certain magnitude and phase angle with respect to M in neighboring voxels. These two quantities are dependent on the relaxation times, spin density, and motion of the protons within the volume element and on details of the MR technique. The phase angle is usually used for determining the spatial location of the MR signals. The magnitude of M in each volume element determines the brightness of each corresponding pixel in the final image.

It is useful to study a simplified model for the intensity of spin–echo signals from tissue:

$$\text{Intensity} = Ne^{-TE/T2}(1 - e^{-TR/T1}) \qquad [7]$$

This model ignores many important factors which affect the spin–echo signal

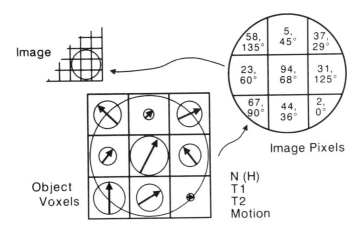

FIG. 11. Relationship between image pixels and object voxels in magnetic resonance imaging.

such as the presence of motion, flow, diffusion, and the technical details of the pulse sequence and imager. Nevertheless, it is very useful for understanding the basis for image contrast.

Note first that the intensity of the signal is proportional to the spin density, and this is true for images with any combination of TR and TE. The dependence of intensity on T2 is governed by the first exponential in this equation and the dependence on T1 is modelled by the terms within the parentheses.

The behavior of the portion of the equation which is within the parentheses is shown in Fig. 2. A spin–echo sequence begins with a 90° RF pulse which tips the magnetization that is parallel to the main magnetic field into the transverse plane. The amount of magnetization which is available for tipping in this manner is dependent on the time that has passed since the previous 90° pulse. Spin–echo sequences with long TR in comparison to the T1 of tissue will have large amounts of magnetization to tip into the transverse plane, whereas short TR values will cause the amount of available longitudinal magnetization to be reduced. When TR is at least three times as long as the T1 of the tissue, then the amount of longitudinal magnetization will be more than 95% of what would be present with an infinite waiting time. If TR is the same as T1 then the magnetization that is available will be approximately 63% of the maximum value. As TR is further reduced, the available magnetization becomes less and less. The latter condition is called a state of partial saturation. Note that a particular repeated spin sequence may cause partial saturation of one tissue with a long T1, whereas some other tissue that has a short T1 may not be partially saturated.

Once the longitudinal magnetization is tipped into the transverse plane by the 90° RF pulse, a spin–echo signal is created at time TE by a 180° RF pulse applied at time TE/2. Equation (7) shows that the intensity or strength of the spin–echo signal depends on an exponential decay function that is governed by the ratio of TE/T2. Clearly, sequences with short echo delay times will produce stronger spin–echoes than those with long TE values in relation to the transverse relaxation time T2. As shown in Fig. 3, tissues with long T2 relaxation times will yield spin–echoes with higher intensity than those with short T2 values, all other factors being equal.

The significance of all of this is that TR is a user selectable parameter that determines the maximum signal that a given tissue will yield (dependent on the rate of growth of longitudinal magnetization, i.e., T1). The selection of TE governs the exponential T2 decay of the potential signal before a spin–echo is created. Given a pair of tissues with different relaxation times, it is possible to select TR and TE in such as way as to either minimize or maximize the intensity difference (contrast) between the two tissues.

Note that equation (7) indicates that if the T1 of a tissue is increased, its spin–echo intensity will be reduced. As shown in Fig. 2, this is because less longitudinal magnetization is available for tipping into the transverse plane and creation of a spin–echo. The reverse condition applies for T2. If the T2 relaxation time of a tissue is increased, its spin–echo intensity will increase because less transverse decay will occur before a spin–echo is formed, as shown in Fig. 3.

T1- AND T2-WEIGHTED SEQUENCES

The concept of T1- and T2-weighted sequences is very useful for selecting sequences and understanding the gray scale of MR images. Consider a hypothetical case in which we wish to determine whether two tissues differ with respect to their T2 relaxation times. This means that it is desirable to select a sequence that is relatively insensitive to differences in T1 but yields intensity differences between tissues with different T2 values that are as large as possible. The first goal can be achieved by selecting a TR time that is long in comparison to the T1 of all of the tissues. Thus, there is enough recovery time between 90° pulses so that full longitudinal magnetization develops in all tissues, regardless of the particular T1 relaxation time. The second goal is facilitated by selecting a TE that is relatively long so that the relative difference in spin–echo intensity between tissues with slow and fast T2 decay is suitably high.

A T2-weighted spin–echo sequence is thus one in which the TR is long in relation to the T1 of the tissues of interest and the TE is also relatively long. The freedom from T1 influence is dependent on TR, and the sensitivity to T2 differences is determined by TE. Although the relative intensity difference between tissues with differing T2 values increases with TE, there is a practical limit to the allowable maximum echo delay time. This is imposed by the fact that the absolute magnitude of the signals decrease with echo delay time so that at some point the ratio of signal-to-noise in the image is degraded so much that further enhancement of relative contrast is useless.

Consider a second case in which we wish to differentiate between tissues on the basis of T1 differences. In order to minimize the intensity differences that would be caused by T2 relaxation, it is necessary to make TE as short as possible. By also selecting a short TR, tissues will be placed in a state of partial saturation, depending on their T1 relaxation time. Tissues with long T1 values will fail to remagnetize as much as those with shorter T1 times, and thus their spin–echo signals will be reduced.

A T1-weighted spin–echo sequence is therefore one with a relatively short TR and short TE. In practice, TE values of less than 20 msec are very difficult to achieve for technical reasons. The extent to which TR can be shortened also has practical limitations because of progressive degradation of signal-to-noise as the time for longitudinal relaxation is reduced. Strongly T1-weighted images can also be generated using IR sequences (see J. Nixon, *this volume*).

The T1- and T2-weighted sequences are very useful for a number of reasons. They allow qualitative recognition of the relaxation time characteristics of lesions in relation to adjacent tissues, which can be very helpful diagnostically. However, their most important role is for combatting the lesion isointensity problem. Many pathological processes, including inflammation, neoplasia, and parenchymal hemorrhage are characterized by parallel increases in both T1 and T2 relaxation times. As already noted, these tend to produce opposite changes in spin–echo intensity, so that for certain combinations of TR and TE, the contrast between a lesion and adjacent normal tissue may be low. Isointensity between tumors and other soft tissue is particularly common with spin–echo sequences that are neither T1- or T2-weighted by the above criteria, especially spin–echo techniques with TR values of 400 to 1,500 and TE values in the range 25 to 40 msec. Figure 12 shows such a situation. The frequency of such problems can be reduced by employing strongly T1- or T2-weighted sequences. In general, the best practice is to image the same area with at least two combinations of TR and TE.

The term "T1-weighted" is frequently misused when it is applied to describe partial saturation (short TR) spin–echo sequences. Although these terms have not been formally defined, it seems clear that in order for a T1-weighted sequence to be useful as such, it must be substantially more sensitive to changes in T1 than to similar percentage changes in T2. Unless this condition is met, lesions that cause simultaneous elevation of T1 and T2 may be missed, and few con-

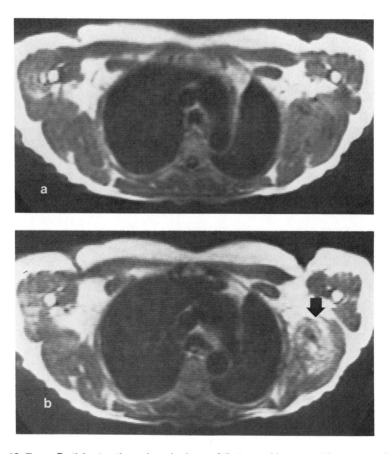

FIG. 12. Top: Partial saturation spin–echo image fails to provide contrast between malignant soft tissue tumor and surrounding muscle. **Bottom:** Tumor is apparent because of contrast provided by T2-weighted spin–echo image (*arrow*).

clusions about relaxation time changes can be made. It is quite difficult to fulfill such a condition with partial saturation spin–echo sequences, because the minimum echo delay time of most imagers still results in substantial T2 dependence.

One way to evaluate the weighting of particular MR imaging techniques is to determine the magnitude and direction of the change in image intensity that would result if the T1 and T2 of a particular tissue is changed by a small amount simultaneously. For example, if T1 and T2 were both increased, then a T1-weighted sequence would register a reduction of intensity and a T2-weighted sequence would show an increase. Mixed or unweighted techniques would yield small or no change of tissue intensity.

Figures 13 and 14 show an example of such an evaluation for spin–echo and IR sequences. In each case, suitable intensity models were used to calculate the percentage change in image intensity that would result from a small percentage increase in T1 and T2 for an ensemble of 25 different tissue relaxation time combinations. In those cases where the intensity increased by a percentage that was at least half of the imposed percentage change in T1 and T2, the sequence was called T2-weighted. Similarly, where the intensity decreased by a percentage that was at least half of the percent change in T1 and T2 it was called T1-weighted. Any sequence that did not yield an intensity change that was more than the arbitrarily chosen limit of half was considered mixed.

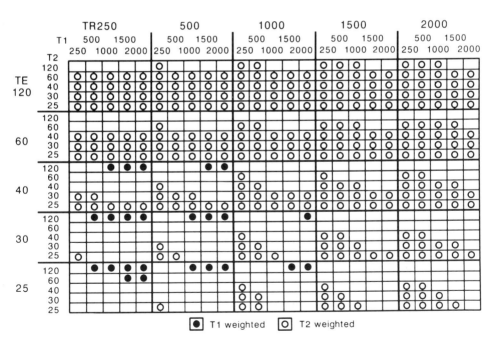

FIG. 13. Map which identifies effective T1- and T2-weighted spin–echo sequences. Each type of sequence is tested against a variety of possible tissue relaxation times.

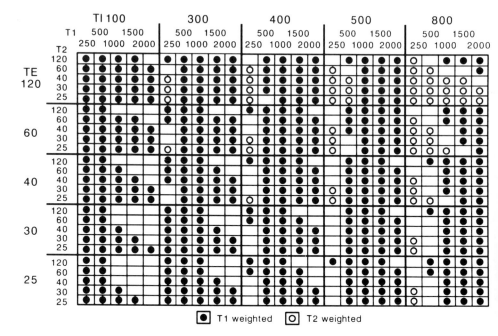

FIG. 14. Map for IR sequences, similar to Fig. 13.

Note that T2-weighted techniques can easily be achieved for most tissues with a variety of spin–echo sequences. On the other hand, it is clearly difficult to obtain a strongly T1-weighted technique using spin–echo sequences unless echo delay times can be drastically shortened. In fact, none of the examined TR and TE combinations provide strongly T1-weighted sequences for most soft tissues. Figure 14 shows that T1-weighted techniques can easily be obtained using IR sequences, even allowing for the spin–echo that is required for data acquisition (IRSE sequence) (45).

The ability to detect lesions in MR imaging is not solely a function of contrast as measured by the relative or absolute intensity differences. Noise is an important additional factor that must be considered. This includes thermal noise and coherent noise (e.g., motion artifacts). Several studies have attempted to find methods to determine specific pulse sequence parameters that optimize the contrast-to-noise ratio for particular lesions (24,31,39). In practice, these approaches have limited value because the relaxation times of pathological and surrounding tissues are rarely known with sufficient precision to make such procedures worthwhile. In addition, optimizing contrast may not be a worthwhile goal because this frequently compromises the clarity of other tissue interfaces. Clearly, the important goal is to simply display the lesion with enough contrast so that it can be detected. This goal is best achieved by imaging with several different MR imaging techniques, at least some of which should be strongly T1- or T2-weighted.

APPROACH FOR SELECTION OF MR IMAGING TECHNIQUES

Certain clinical problems in musculoskeletal MR imaging can serve as examples to clarify the rationale for selecting sequences and interpreting images. These problems include detection of primary soft tissue neoplasms, recurrent tumors after surgery, and identification of hematomas.

As shown elsewhere (T. H. Berquist, "Bone and Soft Tissue Tumors," *this volume*), one of the most successful applications of MR imaging is delineation of soft tissue tumors of the musculoskeletal system. Often these lesions are surrounded by muscle, and it is this situation that we will examine first. We have observed that most malignant lesions have T1 relaxation times that are longer than muscle. Healthy skeletal muscle tissue has a remarkably short T2 relaxation time in comparison to almost any other soft tissue, and certainly its T2 is much shorter than most malignant soft tissue tumors. Given these facts, consider the expected time course of longitudinal magnetization that is shown in Fig. 15a. The longer T1 of tumor means that its longitudinal magnetization will be less than that of muscle, particularly with a short TR such as 500 msec.

Figure 15b shows the time course of the transverse magnetization that would occur after the 180 RF pulse and with a relatively short TR. The shorter T2 of muscle causes its transverse magnetization to decay more quickly than that of the tumor so that the curves cross. Thus, a partial saturation sequence (short TR) with a relatively short TE is likely to display a malignant soft tissue tumor with relatively little contrast. Figure 16a demonstrates such an image in a patient with a malignant schwannoma. In Fig. 15c, the transverse magnetization is traced for the case where a longer TR is used. Note that the starting transverse magnetization is stronger and that the initial difference between tumor and muscle is smaller. With a relatively long echo delay time, the relative intensity difference between tumor and muscle is much greater than in Fig. 15b. Figure 16b shows a corresponding T2-weighted image of the same patient as in Fig. 16a.

The main lesson from this example is that since tumor and muscle differ markedly in their T2 relaxation times, a T2-weighted sequence is able to display the interface with a high degree of contrast. The partial saturation sequence provides a lower degree of contrast in this case because of its mixed response to both T1 and T2 differences.

Tumors are not always completely surrounded by a single tissue, and in these situations several different MR imaging techniques may be necessary to completely delineate the borders of the lesion. A good example of this situation is a follow-up examination in a patient who has previously had a tumor resected from an extremity. Atrophy and fatty infiltration of surrounding muscles is frequently present. Figures 17a and 17b are partial saturation and T2-weighted images from such a patient. Does this patient have recurrent tumor? Figures 18a and 18b are partial saturation and T2-weighted images from a patient with a primary malignant soft tissue tumor in the left popliteal fossa. Can the complete boundaries of the lesion be identified in either image alone?

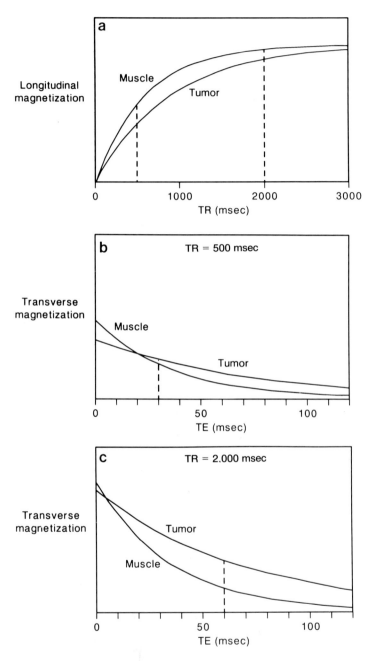

FIG. 15. Typical behavior of longitudinal and transverse magnetization of muscle and tumor in spin–echo sequences. The T2-weighted sequence with long TR and TE provides best contrast.

Adipose tissue has a T1 that is dramatically shorter than almost any other soft tissue as shown in Fig. 7. The T2 relaxation times of fat and tumor can overlap. Figure 19a demonstrates that the longitudinal magnetization that is available in fat is large even with a short TR. In Fig. 19b the transverse magnetization is traced in fat and tumor for a partial saturation sequence. Note that this sequence provides high contrast at short echo delay times. Although transverse magnetization is stronger when the TR is long as shown in Fig. 19c, the contrast between fat and tumor is poor.

Partial saturation sequences therefore are very helpful for differentiating fatty tissue from other tissues. Although they are not particularly T1-weighted, the

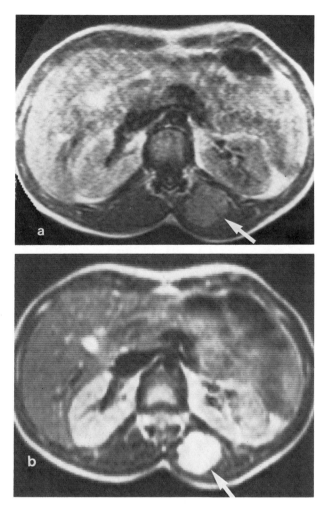

FIG. 16. Partial saturation and T2-weighted spin–echo images of patient with malignant schwannoma (*arrows*), analogous to the situation in Fig. 15.

very short T1 of fat provides sufficient T1 dependent contrast. Figure 17b (T2-weighted image) demonstrates an irregular area of high intensity which could be adipose tissue, but the partial saturation image (Fig. 17a) demonstrates that this is not fat; in fact, this is recurrent tumor. The margins between tumor and adipose tissue are delineated in the partial saturation image in Fig. 18a, but those with muscle are difficult to identify. The T2-weighted image provides just the reverse information.

As described in a previous section, hematomas can have a variety of different appearances because of the unique physical processes that can affect their relaxation times. Some of these are diagnostic. The T1 relaxation times of hematomas may be short at all field strengths due to the proton relaxation enhancement effect of methemoglobin. A second effect that may be characteristic is the selective T2 proton relaxation enhancement produced at high field by deoxyhemoglobin in intact erythrocytes. As demonstrated in Fig. 20, such lesions are of high intensity in both T1- and T2-weighted images at low and medium field strengths. At high field, the selective T2 shortening effect comes into play so that the hematoma may have a very low intensity in both T2-weighted and partial saturation sequences as shown diagrammatically in Fig. 21. A clinical example is shown in Fig. 22.

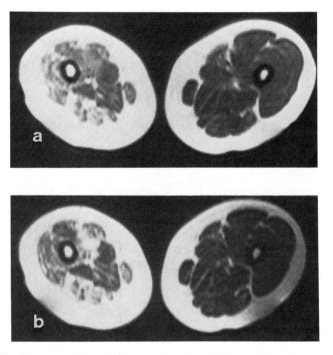

FIG. 17.   Partial saturation and T2-weighted images of a patient with suspected recurrent malignant fibrous histiocytoma. See also Fig. 23.

These examples have shown how it is possible to tailor the contrast of MR imaging sequences by choosing appropriate acquisition parameters. Coupled with a general knowledge of tissue relaxation behavior, this provides a useful qualitative tissue characterization capability, which goes one step beyond morphological imaging.

MISCELLANEOUS TECHNIQUES

A great deal of attention has been directed at the possibility of performing *in vivo* spectroscopy of proton and phosphorus resonances in order to characterize

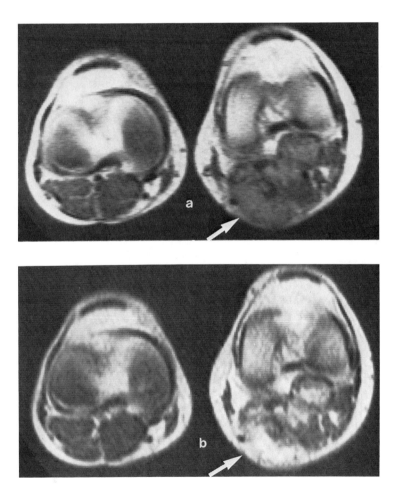

FIG. 18. Partial saturation and T2-weighted sequences are both needed to adequately trace the borders of the malignant tumor in the left popliteal region (*arrows*).

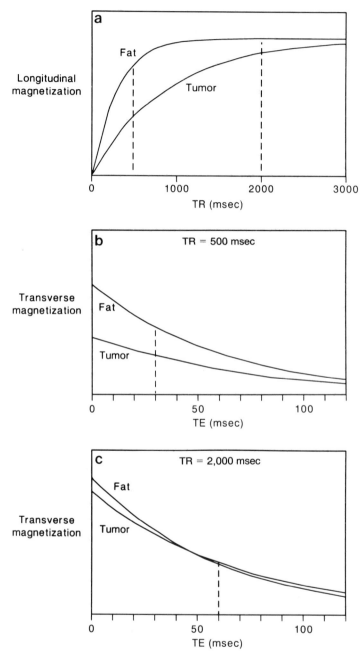

FIG. 19. Contrast between tumor and adipose tissue is most easily achieved with a partial saturation spin–echo sequence with a relatively short TR and TE.

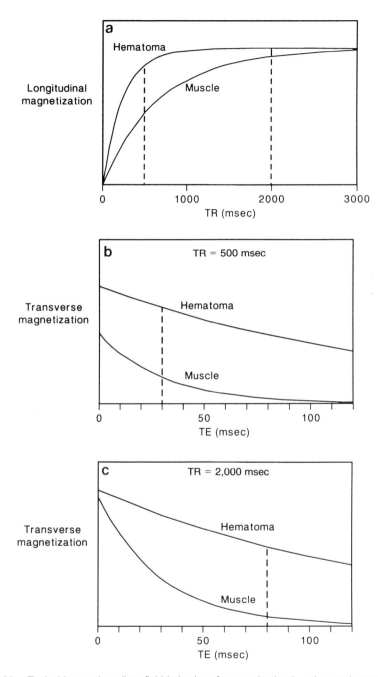

FIG. 20. Typical low and medium field behavior of magnetization in subacute hematoma; **b:** TR = 500 msec; **c:** TR = 2,000 msec.

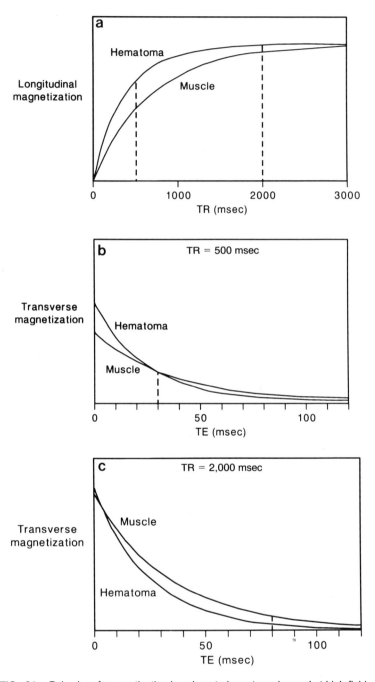

FIG. 21. Behavior of magnetization in subacute hematoma imaged at high field.

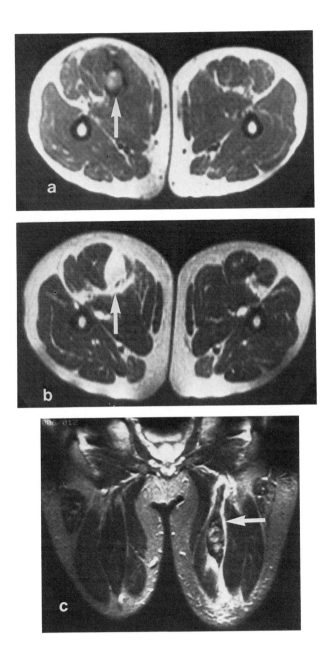

FIG. 22. a: Subacute hematoma imaged at low field (0.15 T) with a strongly T1-weighted sequence. Image demonstrates a halo of low intensity (*arrow*), surrounding a central area of increased intensity. The low intensity is due to prolongation of T1. The area of high intensity is due to T1 shortening caused by a paramagnetic product of oxidative denaturation of hemoglobin. **b:** The hematoma (*arrow*) has a high intensity in T2-weighted images at low field strength because of its long T2 relaxation time. **c:** This coronal T2-weighted image of the same hematoma was acquired on the same date but with a high field imager (1.5 T). The peripheral areas that had the highest intensities with the same sequence in Fig. 22b are of low intensity here because of dramatic T2 shortening at high field.

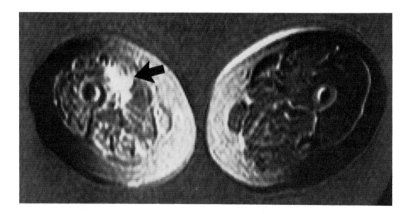

FIG. 23. Subtraction image clearly shows area of combined T1 and T2 prolongation at site of recurrent tumor (*arrow*).

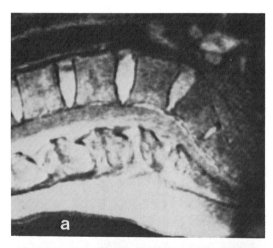

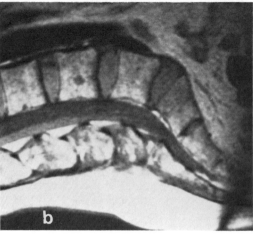

FIG. 24. The pixel intensity in these images depends predominantly on (**a**) water protons and (**b**) fat protons. They were generated by using a simple proton chemical shift imaging approach.

tissue at a biochemical level (18,27,34,35,38,43). These techniques offer potentially exciting prospects, but they remain at an early phase of development.

Many additional techniques for tissue characterization are possible with MR imaging. Some of the simplest ones are most intriguing and seem to be particularly suitable for musculoskeletal problems.

A good example is computation of special-purpose images from standard MR images. Calculated maps of T1, T2, and spin density can be produced, and from them it is possible to generate supplementary images that can depend on any arbitrary function of T1, T2, and N (37). A useful type of image would be one in which increased T1 and T2 relaxation times would both give increased intensity instead of having opposing effects as they do in ordinary images. A simple demonstration of the capability of this type of picture is provided by subtracting the image in Fig. 17a from the image in Fig. 17b. The resultant image has increased intensity in areas of prolonged T2 and prolonged T1 (Fig. 23).

Another example is the development of relatively simple chemical shift techniques that can separate the signals of fat protons from water protons (11) (Fig. 24). These techniques are particularly attractive for certain clinical problems such as characterizing disease of medullary bone (11,48). The opposed-phase

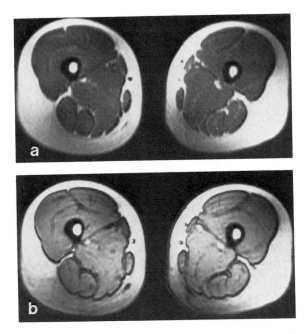

FIG. 25. "In-phase" conventional image (**a**) and "opposed phase" image (**b**) of lower extremeties. Note that a *black line* is interposed at surfaces between tissues that predominantly contain water and those that are fatty. This phase-reversal artifact may be useful in T2 weighted images for delineating small soft tissue structures embedded in adipose tissue, which could otherwise be relatively isointense with fat in conventional in-phase images.

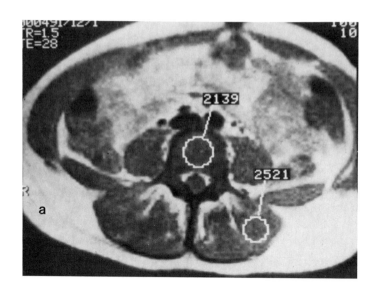

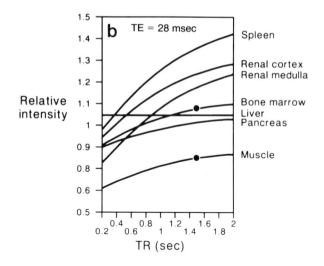

FIG. 26. a: No anatomic lesion is present, yet a relatively gross abnormality is present. This can only be identified by understanding the gray-scale relationships between tissues and how they depend on TR and TE. **b:** A quantitative representation of the normal relative intensities of tissues in spin–echo sequences at a field strength of 0.35 T, based on average relaxation time and spin-density measurements for a large group of patients. Clearly, the normal intensity of skeletal muscle is normally much less than that of medullary bone. As shown in **a**, the intensity of bone marrow in the patient is actually lower than that of paraspinal muscle. This patient has hemosiderosis. Accumulation of hemoglobin breakdown products in bone marrow has shortened its T2 relaxation time.

images which are generated by this technique, although still containing signals from both fat and water protons, seem to have some worthwhile properties beyond the possibility of generating fat and water images. One of these is a narrow, low intensity phase-reversal line which is present at the interfaces between tissues containing predominantly mobile fat and mobile water protons (Fig. 25). This may be helpful for differentiating long-T2, nonfatty tissues from adipose tissue in T2-weighted sequences.

Finally, it should be noted that the quantitative measurements of relative intensity of tissue can be used as a basis for characterization. Figure 26 provides an example.

APPEARANCE OF VASCULAR STRUCTURES IN MR IMAGING

Arteries and veins of varying size can be identified in most musculoskeletal MR images. These vessels are of great intrinsic interest. It is important to define the relationship of major vessels to musculoskeletal tumors if surgery is planned. Many of the primary effects and complications of trauma can affect the vascular supply and drainage of an extremity. Atherosclerosis and deep venous thrombosis are important primary vascular diseases that affect extremities.

For these reasons, it is expected that increasing attention will be paid to the appearance of vascular structures as the diagnostic quality of MR imagery advances. In any case, at the present time it takes only a casual survey of typical MR images to become aware that the appearance of normal arteries and veins can dramatically differ between examinations and from section to section in the same examination. The lumens of vessels may be of low intensity, high intensity,

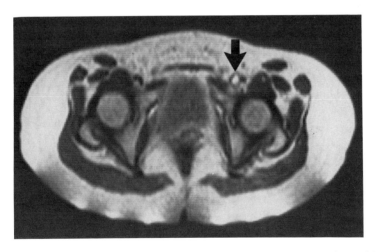

FIG. 27. Thrombosis of left common femoral vein (*arrow*). Note the normal flow void of the femoral artery lateral to the thrombosed vein and the paired-flow voids of the normal right femoral artery and vein.

or mixed intensity. This is disturbing because it hinders reliable identification of such important lesions as venous thrombosis (Figs. 27 and 28).

In order to select examination techniques that facilitate diagnosis of vascular disease and to interpret the images, it is important to have a basic understanding of the physical processes that govern the appearance of moving blood in MR images (1,6,44). For simplicity, this discussion will only consider vessels that are perpendicular to the plane of section.

The signal intensity of flowing blood is governed by three basic processes: saturation, spin phase, and washout effects. Saturation effects (Fig. 29) depend on the fact that the T1 relaxation time of fluid blood is longer than most soft tissues. Thus, the intensity of intravascular blood would be expected to be lower than adjacent tissue if the T1 weighting of a given pulse sequence is sufficient.

The saturation effect is often counteracted by a mechanism called "flow related enhancement" (Fig. 30). This results from flow of blood from outside the image volume in the interval between 90° RF pulses. These fresh spins carry full longitudinal magnetization, because they have not been partially saturated by previous exposure to RF pulses. They can therefore provide more spin–echo signal. This is the main cause of the bright intraluminal signals that are often present in MR images of blood vessels. Naturally, the effect is most pronounced in the sections that are closest to the entry point of the vessel into the image volume.

Two other effects tend to decrease the intensity of flowing blood. One of these is known as the spin dephasing effect. Figures 31a and 31b demonstrate that the volume element corresponding to a single image pixel can be conceptually broken down into smaller volume elements which are called "isochromats." The net magnetization of the entire volume element is the vector sum of the individual magnetizations of the isochromats. If the phase angles of the isochromats are

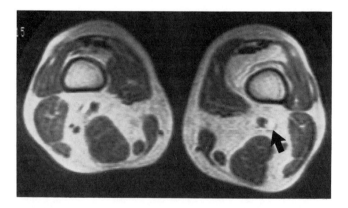

FIG. 28. The lumen of the normal popliteal vein in this image is high intensity due to flow-related enhancement (*arrow*). Thrombosis is not present. Flow void of popliteal artery is located medial to vein. Dissimilar appearance of flowing vessels is due to differing balance of multiple mechanisms that increase and decrease intensity.

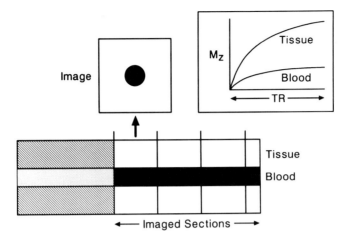

FIG. 29. Saturation effect. Liquid blood has a longer T1 relaxation time than many tissues, especially perivascular fat. Disregarding the effect of flow, it tends to have a lower intensity than surrounding tissue in T1 weighted images because it is more saturated.

not identical, then the magnitude of their vector sum will be reduced. This is the basic principle for spin phase effects. The moving spins in flowing blood are subjected to magnetic field gradients in the course of imaging. These field gradients cause isochromats to accumulate phase differences with respect to stationary spins in tissue. The amount of phase shift depends on the velocity of the individual isochromats and the strength and duration of the field gradients. At the time of

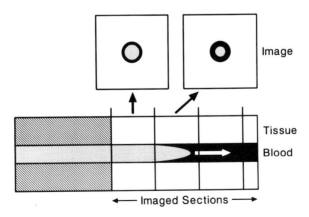

FIG. 30. Flow-related enhancement counteracts the effect of saturation on blood in the vessel lumen. Spins that have not recently been irradiated with RF flow into the plane of section between repetitions. They yield more signal because they are unsaturated. The effect is more pronounced in sections close to the nonirradiated volume.

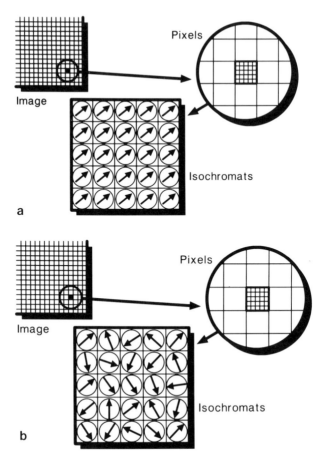

FIG. 31. The contents of a voxel can be conceptually divided into smaller elements called isochromats. The spin–echo signal from each isochromat is a vector quantity, having a magnitude and phase (direction). If the phase angles of most isochromats are similar (**a**), then the vectors add constructively. If varied phase angles are present (**b**), then the net signal from the volume element will be reduced.

the first spin–echo, the magnetization isochromats with varying phase angles add together in an incoherent fashion so that signal intensity is reduced.

This situation is shown schematically for laminar flow on the right of Fig. 32. Figure 33b is a graph of the phase angle of three different isochromats flowing through the same field gradient. Note that the polarity of the phase errors is reversed by the 180° RF pulse. At the time of the first spin–echo, the phase angles of the isochromats are different, so that these and the other elements of the voxel do not add coherently and the intensity of the spin–echo signal is reduced. This explanation suggests that velocity differences between isochromats are the main cause of spin phase effects, divergent phase angles, but shear is

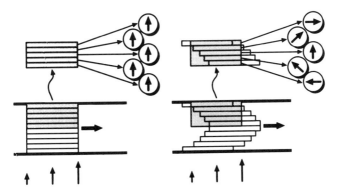

FIG. 32. Dephasing effect. **Left:** "Plug flow," is a model for flow that assumes that the velocity of fluid is the same near the center of the lumen as it is at the sides. Thus, each isochromat has the same velocity. The *vertical arrows* along the base of the vessel represent the strength of the local magnetic field at each point. This gradient causes the phase angle of each isochromat to change as it flows along the vessel, but since the velocities are identical, the phase angles of all the isochromats in the volume element will be the same at the time of the spin–echo. **Right:** "Laminar flow," is a situation in which the velocity has a parabolic profile across the lumen of the vessel. In this case, the phase errors accumulated by isochromats as they flow through the magnetic field gradient are variable because the velocities are different. Thus, the net signal intensity from a voxel is reduced at the time of spin–echo creation because the isochromats do not add constructively. This has been called the "dephasing effect."

actually not required to cause intensity loss in an imaging situation, as described in the next paragraph.

The case of plug flow, where all of the isochromats move at the same velocity, is shown on the left in Fig. 32. The corresponding spin phase graph in Fig. 33a shows that although the phase angles of isochromats at the leading and trailing edges of the plug initially diverge, they reconverge at the time of the first spin–echo. Although there is no phase divergence to reduce intensity in this case, there is a net phase error for the entire volume element. If flow is pulsatile, the process of imaging and averaging will result in a reduction of the intensity of the corresponding image pixel, because individual phase encoding views and averages will obtain a random phase angle from the volume element. This plug flow mechanism may actually be a more important cause of first echo intensity loss in clinical images than the velocity shear mechanism described above.

The dephasing effects can reduce the intensity of blood in first echo (and other odd numbered echoes in multiple spin–echo sequences) masking any flow-related enhancement which may have been present. Even-echo-rephasing is a striking phenomenon which can counteract the dephasing effects of gradients so that intensity is restored in even-numbered echoes (Fig. 34). This depends on a peculiar property of even-numbered echoes in multiple spin–echo sequences. Under certain circumstances, the even-numbered 180° pulses may at least partially correct the phase errors that are induced by flow through gradients. This is schematically shown for the simulations of plug and laminar flow in Figs. 33a and 33b.

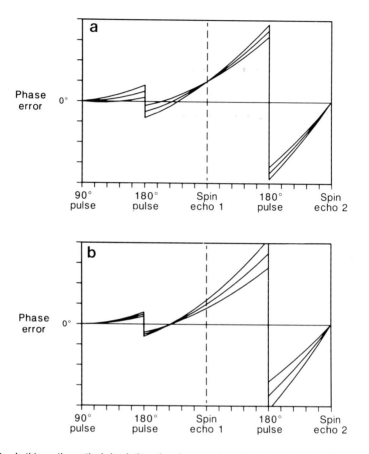

FIG. 33. In this mathematical simulation, the phase angles of three isochromats that are flowing through a magnetic field gradient are graphed versus time for a double-spin–echo sequence. The phase angle of stationary tissue is zero throughout the sequence so that the phase angles of the isochromats can be regarded as phase errors if they are not zero. **a:** Plug flow. Each isochromat has the same velocity, but has a slightly different starting point along the vessel. Note that at the time of the first spin–echo, the accumulated phase angle of each of the three isochromats is identical and nonzero. The intensity of the net spin–echo signal from a voxel in this case will be the same as if the fluid was stationary, but the phase angle will be different from that of stationary tissue. In practice, blood flow is variable, and if the spin–echo experiment is repeated several times, the phase angle of each acquistion will be different. Thus, with averaging, the mean signal will be reduced. The simulation shows the surprising result that at the time of the second spin–echo, the phase angles of the isochromats are not only identical but the same as stationary tissue. This has been called the "rephasing phenomenon." **b:** Laminar flow. Each of the three isochromats in the simulation is flowing at a slightly different rate. At the time of the first spin–echo, the phase angles are nonzero and different. This phase dispersion means that the signals from each isochromat will not add constructively and that the net spin–echo signal will be reduced. Following the first echo, the phase angles of the isochromats continue to diverge, but the second 180° pulse has the effect of restoring phase coherence at the time of the second spin–echo. The rephasing phenomenon can cause the signal intensity that was lost in the first echo due to phase dispersion to be restored in the second echo.

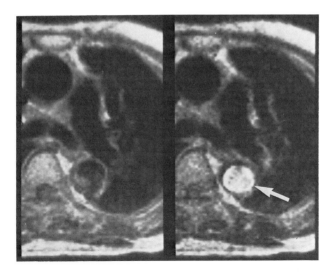

FIG. 34. An example of first-echo dephasing and second-echo rephasing in the descending aorta (*arrow*). The signal intensity observed in the lumen of a vessel is affected by the summation of flow effects. In the 28-msec first-echo image, unsaturated spins from distant points outside the images volume are present within the lumen of the descending aorta, but flow related enhancement is not observed because the intensity is reduced by the dephasing phenomenon. This flow related enhancement is "uncovered" in the second-echo image because of the rephasing effect, which corrects the phase dispersion which was present at the time of the first echo.

The most important mechanism that reduces the MR image intensity of flowing blood has not yet been described here. This is the washout effect, shown in Fig. 35. Protons must receive both 90° and 180° RF pulses in order to yield a spin–echo signal. In most imagers, these pulses are slice selective so that their effects are spatially limited to the confines of imaged sections. Flowing protons that

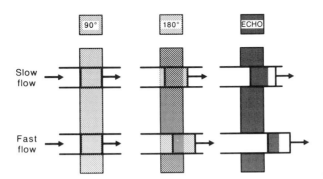

FIG. 35. Ilustration of the "washout effect." Those flowing spins that move out of the section in the time between 90° and 180° pulses will not yield a spin–echo signal. The amount of signal loss due to washout increases with flow velocity. With very fast flow, all of the blood in the segment of lumen may be replaced so that the spin–echo signal will be zero. The minimum velocity that replaces all spins in such a fashion is called the cutoff velocity.

escape the plane of section in the time interval between 90 and 180° RF pulses will not produce a signal. This establishes a cutoff velocity for blood flow, above which no intraluminal signal can be present. This velocity can be calculated by dividing the section thickness by time interval between the 90 and 180° RF pulses.

Based on the preceding discussion, it is clear that intraluminal blackness (flow voids) in blood vessels can be promoted by enlarging the volume that is irradiated with RF in order to minimize flow-related enhancement, employing odd-numbered echoes to allow dephasing and longer echo delay times to allow washout to occur. Many different flow effects can be observed in MR imaging, but the principles described above can be used to explain most of them.

REFERENCES

1. Axel, L. (1984): Blood flow effects in magnetic resonance imaging. *A. J. R.,* 143:1157–1166.
2. Beall, P. T., Amtey, S. R., and Kasturi, S. R. (1984): *NMR Data Handbook for Biomedical Applications,* Table 9.10. Pergamon, New York.
3. Bloemberger, E. M., Purcell, E. M., and Pound, R. V. (1948): Relaxation effects in nuclear magnetic resonance absorption. *Phys. Rev.,* 73:679–712.
4. Bottomley, P. A., Foster, T. H., Argersinger, R. E., and Pfeifer, L. M. (1984): A review of normal tissue hydrogen NMR relaxation times and relaxation mechanisms from 1–100 MHz: dependence on tissue type, NMR frequency. *Med. Phys.,* 11:425–448.
5. Bradley, W. G., and Schmidt, P. G. (1985): Effect of methemoglobin formation on the appearance of subarachnoid hemorrhage. *Radiology,* 156:99–103.
6. Bradley, W. G., and Waluch, V. (1985): Blood flow: magnetic resonance imaging. *Radiology,* 154:443–450.
7. Brasch, R. C. (1983): Work in progress: methods of contrast enhancement for NMR imaging and potential applications. *Radiology,* 147:781–788.
8. Brasch, R. C., Wesbey, G. E., Gooding, C. A., and Koerper, M. A. (1984): Magnetic resonance imaging of transfusional hemosiderosis complicating thalasemia major. *Radiology,* 150:767–771.
9. Crooks, L. E., Arakawa, M., Hoenninger, J., McCarten, B., Watts, J., and Kaufman, L. (1984): Magnetic resonance imaging: effects of magnetic field strength. *Radiology,* 151:127–133.
10. De Vre, R. M. (1984): Biomedical implications of the relaxation behavior of water related to NMR imaging. *Br. J. Radiol.,* 57:955–976.
11. Dixon, W. T. (1984): Simple proton spectroscopic imaging. *Radiology,* 153:189–194.
12. Dooms, G. C., Fisher, M. R., Hricak, H., and Higgins, C. B. (1985): MR imaging of intramuscular hemorrhage. *J. Comput. Assist. Tomogr.,* 9:908–913.
13. Dooms, G. C., Hricak, H., Moseley, M. E., Bottles, K., Fisher, M., and Higgins, C. B. (1985): Characterization of lymphadenopathy by magnetic resonance relaxation times: preliminary results. *Radiology,* 155:691–697.
14. Ehman, R. L., Kjos, B. O., Hricak, H., Brasch, R. C., and Higgins, C. B. (1985): Relative intensity of abdominal organs in magnetic resonance images. *J. Comput. Assist. Tomogr.,* 9:315–319
15. Ehman, R. L., McNamara, M. T., Brasch, R. C., Felmlee, J. P., Gray, J. E., and Higgins, C. B. (1986): Influence of physiological motion on the appearance of tissue in MRI. *Radiology (in press).*
16. Ehman, R. L., McNamara, M. T., Pallack, M., Hricak, H., and Higgins, C. B. (1984): Magnetic resonance imaging with respiratory gating: techniques and advantages. *A. J. R.,* 143:1175–1182.
17. Farrar, T. C., and Becker, E. D. (1971): *Pulse and Fourier Transform NMR: Introduction to Theory and Methods.* Academic Press, New York.
18. Frahm, J., Haase, A., Hanicke, W., Matthaei, D., Hartwin, B., and Helzel, T. (1985): Chemical shift selective MR imaging using a whole body magnet. *Radiology,* 156:441–444.

19. Fullerton, G. D., Cameron, I. L., Hunter, K., and Fullerton, H. (1985): Proton magnetic resonance relaxation behavior of whole muscle with fatty inclusions. *Radiology,* 155:727–730.
20. Fullerton, G. D., Cameron, I. L., and Ord, V. A. (1984): Frequency dependence of magnetic resonance spin-lattice relaxation of protons in biological materials. *Radiology,* 151:135–138.
21. Fullerton, G. D., Potter, J. L., and Dornbluth, N. C. (1982): NMR relaxation of protons in tissues and other macromolecular water solutions. *Magnetic Resonance Imaging,* 1:209–228.
22. Gomori, J. M., Grossman, R. I., Goldberg, H. I., Zimmerman, R. A., and Bilaniuk, L. T. (1985): Intracranial hematomas: imaging by high field MR. *Radiology,* 157:87–93.
23. Hazelwood, C. F. (1979): A view of the significance and understanding of the physical properties of cell-associated water. In: *Cell Associated Water,* edited by W. Drost-Hansen and J. Clegg, pp. 165–260. Academic Press, New York.
24. Hendrick, R. E., Nelson, T. R., and Hendee, W. R. (1984): Optimizing tissue contrast in magnetic resonance imaging. *Magnetic Resonance Imaging,* 2:193–204.
25. Herfkins, R., Davis, P. L., Crooks, L. E., Kaufman, L., Price, D., Miller, T., and Margulis, A. (1981): Nuclear magnetic resonance imaging of the abnormal live rat and correlations with tissue characteristics. *Radiology,* 141:211–218.
26. Johnson, G. A., Herfkins, R. J., and Brown, M. A. (1985): Tissue relaxation time: in vivo field dependence. *Radiology,* 156:805–810.
27. Joseph, P. M. (1985): A spin echo chemical shift MR imaging technique. *J. Comput. Assist. Tomogr.,* 9:651–658.
28. Joseph, P. M., and Axel, L. (1984): Potential problems with selective pulses in NMR imaging systems. *Med. Phys.,* 11:772–777.
29. Kjos, B. O., Ehman, R. L., and Brant-Zawadzki, M. (1985): Reproducibility of t1 and t2 relaxation times calculated from routine MR imaging sequences: phantom study. *A. J. N. R.,* 6:277–283.
30. Kjos, B. O., Ehman, R. L., Brant-Zawadzki, M., Kelly, W. M., Norman, D., and Newton, T. H. (1985): Reproducibility of relaxation times and spin density calculated from routine MR imaging sequences: clinical study of the CNS. *A. J. N. R.,* 6:271–276.
31. Kurtz, D., and Dwyer, A. (1984): Isosignal contours and signal gradients as an aid to choosing MRI imaging techniques. *J. Comput. Assist. Tomogr.,* 8:819–828.
32. Lee, J. K., Dixon, W. T., Ling, D., Levitt, R. G., and Murphy, W. A. (1984): Fatty infiltration of the liver: demonstration by proton spectroscopic imaging. *Radiology,* 153:195–201.
33. McSweeney, M. B., Small, W. C., Cerny, V., et al. (1984): Magnetic resonance imaging in the diagnosis of breast disease: use of transverse relaxation times. *Radiology,* 153:741–744.
34. Newman, R. J., Bore, P. J., Chan, L., Gadian, D. G., et al. (1982): Nuclear magnetic resonance studies of forearm muscle in Duchenne dystrophy. *Br. Med. J. [Clin. Res.],* 284:1072–1074.
35. Nidecker, A. C., Muller, S., Aue, W. P. (1985): Extremity bone tumors: evaluation by p-31 spectroscopy. *Radiology,* 157:167–174.
36. Ohtomo, K., Itai, Y., Furui, S., et al. (1985): Hepatic tumors: differentiation by transverse relaxation time (t2) of MR resonance imaging. *Radiology,* 155:421–423.
37. Ortendahl, D. A., Hylton, N., Kaufman, L., Watts, J. C., Crooks, L. E., and Mills, C. M. (1984): Star analytical tools for magnetic resonance imaging. *Radiology,* 153:479–488.
38. Pykett, I. L., and Rosen, B. R. (1983): Nuclear magnetic resonance in vivo proton chemical shift imaging. *Radiology,* 149:197–201.
39. Richardson, M. L., Amparo, E. G., Gillespy, T., Helms, C. A., Demas, B. E., and Genant, H. K. (1985): Theoretical considerations for optimizing intensity differences between primary musculoskeletal tumors and normal tissue with spin echo MRI. *Invest. Radiol.,* 20:492–497.
40. Schmidt, H. C., Tscholakoff, D., Hricak, H., and Higgins, C. B. (1985): MR image contrast and relaxation times of solid tumors in the chest, abdomen, and pelvis. *J. Comput. Assist. Tomogr.,* 9:738–748.
41. Swenson, S. J., Keller, P. L., Berquist, T. H., Mcleod, R. A., and Stephens, D. H. (1985): Magnetic resonance imaging of hemorrhage. *A. J. R.,* 145:921–927.
42. Thulborn, K. R., Waterton, J. C., Matthews, P. M., and Radda G. K. (1982): Oxygenation dependence of the transverse relaxation time of water protons in whole blood at high field. *Biochemica et Biophysica Acta,* 714:265–270.
43. Vock, P., Hoppeler, H., Hartl, W., and Fritschy, P. (1985): Combined use of MRI and MRS by

whole body magnets in studying skeletal muscle morphology and metabolism. *Invest. Radiol.,* 20:486–491.
44. Wehrli, F. W., MacFall, J. R., Axel, L., Shutts, D., Glover, G. H., and Herfkins, R. J. (1984): Approaches to in-plane and out-of-plane flow imaging. *Noninvasive Medical Imaging,* 1:127–136.
45. Wehrli, F. W., MacFall, J. R., Shutts, D., Breger, R., and Herfkens, R. J. (1984): Mechanisms of contrast in NMR imaging. *J. Comput. Assist. Tomogr.,* 8:369–380.
46. Wesbey, G. E., Moseley, M., and Ehman, R. L. (1984): Translational molecular self-diffusion in magnetic resonance imaging: effects on observed spin-spin relaxation. *Invest. Radiol.,* 19:484–490.
47. Wesbey, G. E., Moseley, M., and Ehman, R. L. (1984): Translational molecular self-diffusion in magnetic resonance imaging: measurement of the self-diffusion coefficient. *Invest. Radiol.,* 19:491–498.
48. Wismer, G. L., Rosen, B. R., Buxton, R., Stark, D. D., and Brady, T. J. (1985): Chemical shift imaging of bone marrow: preliminary experience. *A. J. R.,* 145:1031–1037.
49. Zimmer, W. D., Berquist, T. H., Mcleod, R. A., et al. (1985): Bone tumors: magnetic resonance imaging versus computed tomography. *Radiology,* 155:709–718.

Technical Considerations in Magnetic Resonance Imaging

Thomas H. Berquist

Mayo Medical School, and Department of Diagnostic Radiology,
Mayo Clinic, Rochester, Minnesota 55905

Magnetic resonance (MR) imaging is an excellent technique for evaluation of the musculoskeletal system (2,6,10). Respiratory motion, a significant problem in the chest and upper abdomen, is generally not a problem in the pelvis and extremities. Images can be obtained in the coronal, sagittal, and transaxial planes. Also, soft tissue contrast is superior to computed tomography (CT) and conventional imaging techniques. Table 1 lists the MR image appearance of musculoskeletal tissues in order of decreasing signal intensity (2,6,10,11). Fat and medullary bone have the highest signal intensity and appear white on MR images (Table 1). The signal intensity of articular cartilage is between muscle and medullary bone. It has been suggested that the different image appearance of articular and meniscal cartilage is probably due to variations in the types of collagen and water content in these structures (6). The water content of articular cartilage is higher (75 to 80%) than menisci. Menisci, ligaments, and tendons appear black

TABLE 1. *Signal intensity of musculoskeletal tissues*

Signal intensity	Tissue
Highest (white)	Fat
	Medullary bone
Gray	Articular cartilage
Intermediate intensity	Muscle
Low intensity (black)	Blood vessels[a]
	Ligaments, tendons
	Menisci
	Cortical bone

[a] Normally flowing blood gives no signal. The appearance of vessels may vary with changes in flow and multiecho sequences.

65

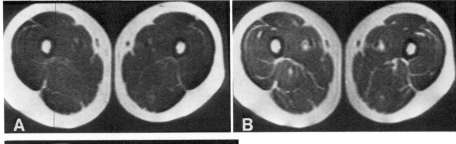

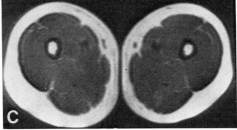

FIG. 1. Transaxial images of the thighs using inversion recovery with a TI 500 and TR 1500 (**A**), spin–echo with a TE 60 and TR 2000 (**B**), and partial saturation with TE 30 and TR 133 (**C**).

on MR images. These structures are composed of predominantly Type I collagen (articular cartilage is Type II) and contain less water (6). Blood vessels also appear black if flow is normal. However, signal intensity in vascular structures may increase due to abnormal flow or if thrombosis has occurred. Increased signal intensity in vessels also occurs due to artifact and with multislice, multiecho sequences (see R. L. Ehman, *this volume*). Cortical bone is white on CT images and often causes significant streak (beam hardening) artifacts. Cortical bone is black on MR images, and there is no artifact. This allows more complete evaluation of adjacent soft tissues (Fig. 4). The signal intensity of normal tissues does not vary significantly when using common pulse sequence [spin–echo with long echo time (TE) and repetition time (TR) and short TE and TR, or inversion recovery (IR)] (6) (Fig. 1).

MR imaging examinations must be conducted differently than conventional radiographic or CT examinations. Patient selection, positioning, coil selection, and pulse sequences must all be considered to optimize information on the images.

PATIENT SELECTION

MR images are produced using a static magnetic field, magnetic gradients, and radiofrequency (RF) pulses (see J. Nixon, *this volume*). There is no ionizing radiation. To date, no biological hazards have been identified at the currently used field strengths [≤2 T (tesla)] (14,16).

The MR imaging gantry is more confining than a conventional fluoroscopic unit or CT scanner. Patients are positioned in the center of the cylindrical magnet chamber during the examination (Fig. 2). Despite this apparent drawback we

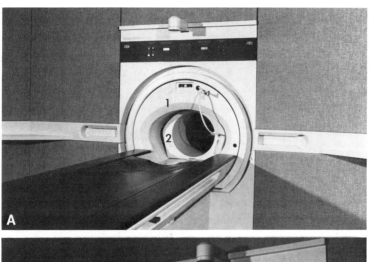

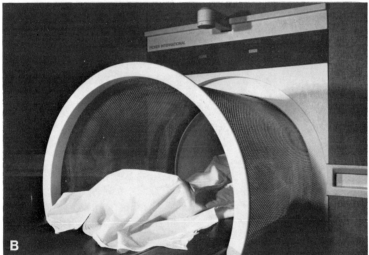

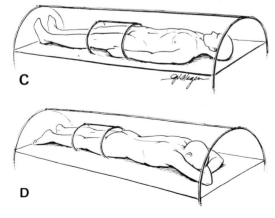

FIG. 2. Resistive MR imager with the body (**1**) and head (**2**) coils in position (**A**). When the patient is examined (**B**) the RF shield is pulled forward. The position of the patient and corset coil for examination of the thighs is illustrated in both the supine (**C**) and prone (**D**) positions.

noted problems with claustrophobia in only 2 to 3% of our first 4,500 patients. Patients with claustrophobic tendencies seem to tolerate MR examinations more readily if they are in the prone position. If necessary, mild sedation with oral valium may be helpful. Patient size can also be a limiting factor. Body coils are usually only about 53 × 35 cm which may make imaging of large patients difficult or impossible.

The patient's clinical status must be considered. Patients with significant pain or inability to maintain the necessary positions may not be able to tolerate the potentially lengthy examinations. Premedication with valium or demerol may be useful in these cases. Initially there was concern that severely ill patients requiring cardiac monitoring and respiratory support could not be examined. Remember ferromagnetic anesthesia equipment cannot be moved into the magnet room or near the gantry without affecting the images. Our experience shows that these patients can be monitored successfully without interfering with image quality. Initially we studied 20 patients requiring cardiac and respiratory support. Patients were monitored with a blood pressure cuff with plastic connectors, an Aneuroid Chest Bellows (Coulbourn Instruments, Allentown, Pennsylvania) for respiratory rate, and a Hewlett-Packard ECG telemetry system (Hewlett Packard, Waltham, Massachusetts). The respiratory rate and ECG were monitored on a Saturn monitor (Spacelabs Inc., Chatsworth, California). Certain problems were encountered during the study. RF pulses caused ECG artifacts (Fig. 3), especially if short repetition times were used. This problem was overcome by using a Doppler system to monitor the pulse during the imaging sequences. Satisfactory monitoring was achieved in all patients, and equipment used did not affect image quality (13).

Magnetic fields may affect certain metal implants and electrical devices. In most situations the exact chemical structure of the implant cannot be determined (8). Fortunately, early efforts to determine which implants may be potentially dangerous to the patient or affect image quality have been successful (2,3,8,11,12,17). Synchronous pacemakers convert to the asynchronous mode when placed in MR imagers. The pacemaker power pack may torque in the

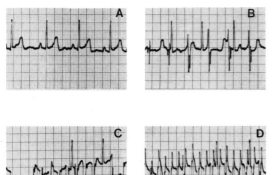

FIG. 3. Effect of RF pulsing on ECG monitoring. (A) No RF in use. RF pulses with 500 (B), 200 (C), and 166 (D) msec intervals. (From Roth et al., ref. 13, with permission.)

magnetic field. In addition, significant image degradation may occur if the power pack is in the region being examined (12). Numerous heart valves have been studied at field strengths of 0.35 and 1.5 T. The artifacts created were negligible, and it was concluded that patients with prosthetic valves could be safely imaged (17).

Most surgical clips at our institution are nonferromagnetic. However, a significant number of aneurysm clips (16/21) are ferromagnetic, and torquing can be demonstrated in a magnetic environment (11). Therefore, patients with aneurysm clips or pacemakers are currently not examined.

Manufacturers of orthopedic appliances (plates, screws, joint prostheses, etc.) generally use high-grade stainless steel, cobalt–chromium, titanium, or multiphase alloys. These materials are usually not ferromagnetic but may contain minimal quantities of iron impurities. All of the orthopedic appliances at our institution have been tested for magnetic properties (torque in the magnet) and heating. No heating or magnetic response could be detected (2). Davis et al. (3) also studied the effects of RF pulses and changing magnetic fields on metal clips and prosthesis. No heating could be detected with small amounts of metal. Heating was demonstrated with two adjacent hip prostheses in a saline medium. However, it was concluded that metal heating in patients should not be a problem even with large prostheses (3,8).

Metal materials cause significant artifact on CT images (2,3,9). Nonferromagnetic materials cause areas of no signal but less artifact on MR images (Fig. 4). The degree of artifact is dependent on the size and configuration of the metal. When imaging a hip prosthesis, more artifact is created by the large irregular head and neck region than the more regular and smaller femoral stem (Fig. 4). There is also more artifact from metal screws and Harrington rods (2,8) (Fig. 5). This may be due to the irregular contour (threads and ridges), screw position, or increased amounts of ferromagnetic impurities. The latter problem is demonstrated in Fig. 6. There are only two screws, yet there is a significant amount of artifact. There are also artifacts in the region of old pin tracts. The radiograph (Fig. 6A) does not demonstrate metal in these old pin tracts. Even small amounts of ferromagnetic materials can cause significant artifact (11). This fact, coupled with histologic evidence of metal debris in histiocytes around screw tracts, suggests that small amounts of ferromagnetic material are present in some screws used for internal fixation. A fibrohistiocytic response normally occurs around these screws if left in place for a significant length of time (months). This phenomenon may allow artifact to occur even though no significant metal can be detected on routine radiographs (Fig. 7).

External fixation devices may be bulky, but most are not ferromagnetic (Fig. 8) as the materials are similar to those used in internal fixateurs. Magnetic properties can be easily checked with a hand-held magnet prior to the MR examination. Coil selection may be restricted due to the size of these fixation systems. This can result in a decreased signal-to-noise ratio and reduce image quality. However, most patients can be examined using head or body coils.

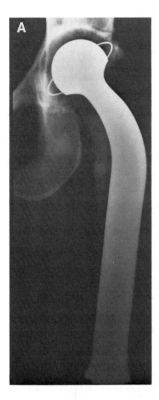

FIG. 4. Radiograph of a custom total hip arthroplasty (**A**) demonstrating the large amount of metal in the hip and femur. The transaxial CT image through the femoral heads (**B**) is degraded by metal artifact. The MR image (**C**) at the same level is less degraded though there is some distortion due to the size and configuration of the metal. In the region of the small smooth femoral stem there is still significant artifact on the CT image (**D**), but no artifact on the MR image (**E**).

Early experience with metal implants at low and high field strength (0.15 to 1.5 T) shows that artifact is slightly more obvious at higher field strengths (8). Evaluation of patients with casts and bulky dressings (Robert–Jones, etc.) is also possible with MR imaging. We have not detected any reduction in image quality because of these materials.

PATIENT POSITIONING

Patient positioning considerations include size, body part, and expected examination time. The patient should be studied with the most closely coupled coil possible to achieve the maximum signal-to-noise ratio and best spatial resolution (2,5) (Fig. 9). Signal-to-noise ratios may be increased four to six times with a limb coil compared to the head and body coils (5). Examination of the trunk, pelvis, and upper thighs is usually performed in the body coil or closer fitting corset coil. The head coil can occasionally be used in thin patients and children. The knees, legs, and foot and ankle can be examined in the knee coil (Fig. 9B). Small circular or flat coils are also available with high field (1.5 T) magnets and should be used when they fit the clinical setting (Fig. 10).

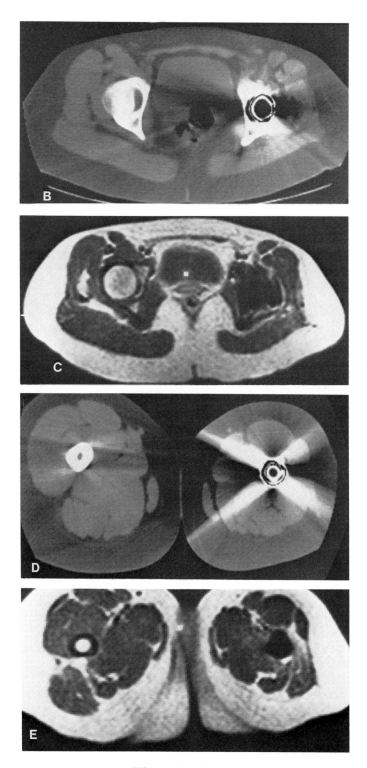

FIG. 4. (Continued.)

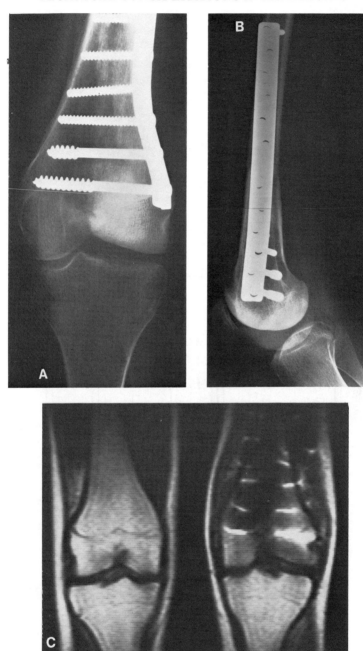

FIG. 5. AP (**A**) and lateral (**B**) radiographs of the distal femur with a large plate and multiple metallic screws. The corresponding coronal (**C**) and sagittal (**D**) MR images show more artifact than in Fig. 4. This may be related to the position, number, and irregularity of the screws. The amount of ferromagnetic impurity is probably also greater in the screws. The transaxial view (**E**) is also affected by the artifact, but the soft tissues can still be adequately evaluated.

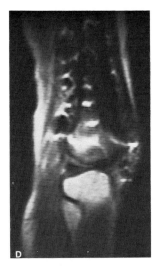
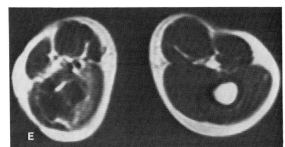

FIG. 5.   (Continued.)

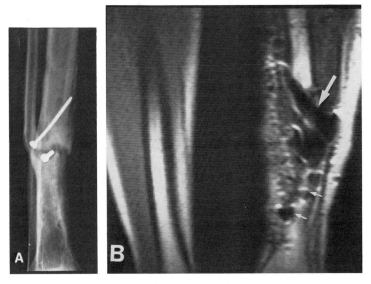

FIG. 6.   Radiograph (A) demonstrating an old ununited fracture of the tibia with multiple pin tracts above and below the fracture. The MR image (B) demonstrates considerably more artifact than would be expected from these two screws (*large arrow*). Note the numerous artifacts (*small arrows*) in the pin tracts.

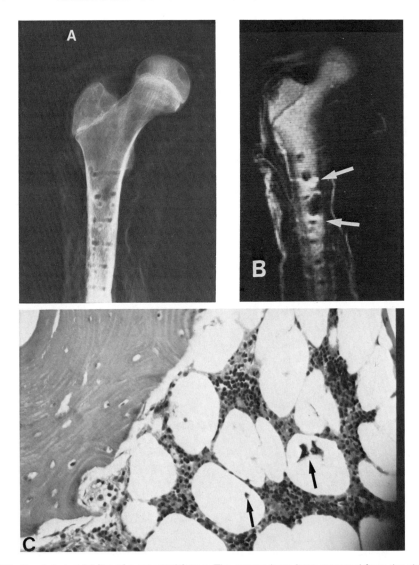

FIG. 7.   A: Industrial film of a resected femur. The screws have been removed from the shaft and there is no evidence of residual metal. **B:** MR image of the femur (TE 30, TR 500) shows multiple artifacts (*arrows*) in the pin tracts. **C:** Histologic specimen of the pin tract demonstrating metal debris (*arrows*). (Courtesy of Les Wold, M.D., Department of Surgical Pathology, Mayo Clinic, Rochester, Minnesota.)

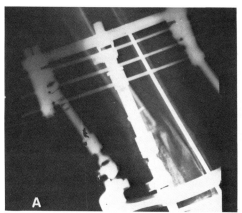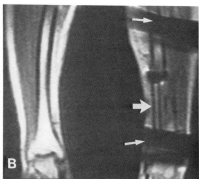

FIG. 8. A: Radiograph taken in an Ace–Fischer external fixation device following placement of a fibular graft. The fixation device causes areas of no signal (*small white arrows*) on the coronal MR image (**B**), but the fibular graft (*large white arrow*) is well demonstrated.

If comparison with the opposite extremity is needed the head coil (Fig. 8D) is usually used. Patients can be positioned prone or supine depending on the indication for the study. If the posterior soft tissues are being examined the prone position should be used to prevent tissue distortion (Fig. 11). Also, when two extremities are being examined, vertical phase encoding is preferred. If there is motion from pain in one extremity the artifact created will affect both legs if horizontal encoding is used (Fig. 12). The normal angles of the spine and extremities must be considered in planning the examination (Fig. 13). Coronal and sagittal images do not necessarily mean that partial volume effects are a less significant problem than with axial CT images (Figs. 13B and 13C). This must be kept in mind when evaluating the extent of disease processes in the coronal and sagittal planes.

Imaging of the upper extremities has been more difficult due to problems with patient positioning and the reduced tissue volume, especially in the hand and wrist. If conventional coils (head and body) are used to examine the forearm or wrist, the filling factor is reduced resulting in less signal and increased noise. Thus, the images are frequently suboptimal. This problem can be overcome by using small closely coupled coils. Surface coil images using high field (1.5 T) magnets now provide dramatic improvement in image detail (Figs. 14 and 15). These coils improve the signal-to-noise ratio significantly (1,5,15). With noncircumferential surface coils (flat or incomplete circle) the depth of view is limited. As a rule, the depth of view of a flat coil is approximately one-half the diameter or width of the coil (5). In addition, these coils are most effective when centered in the magnetic field. When these coils are off-center the image quality and choice of the size of field of views are limited. Therefore, position for examination of the forearm, elbow, and hand and wrist generally requires the patient to position the arm above the head (Fig. 16). This position is uncomfortable and

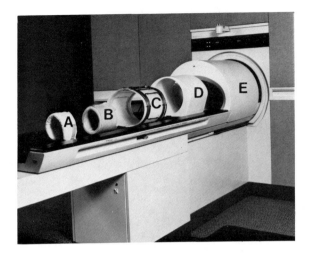

FIG. 9. Illustration of coils used with a resistive system: (*A*) closely coupled saddle coil (neck, peripheral extremities); (*B*) knee coil (knee, peripheral extremities); (*C*) corset coil (trunk, thighs, shoulders); (*D*) head coil (thin patients, upper and lower extremities); (*E*) body coil (thighs and trunk).

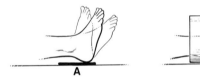

FIG. 10. Illustration of coils [flat (**A**) and circumferential (**B**)] for examination of the ankle. The position of the foot is more restricted by a coil which surrounds the foot. This may change the degree of tension on the Achilles and other tendons which can affect their image appearance.

FIG. 11. Illustration of the calves in the supine and prone position. The posterior soft tissues are compressed in the supine position.

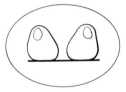
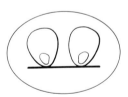

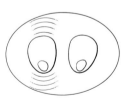
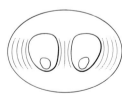

FIG. 12. Illustration of motion artifact of calves with the patient prone. If the right extremity is moving slightly the artifact affects both legs with horizontal but only the moving leg with vertical encoding.

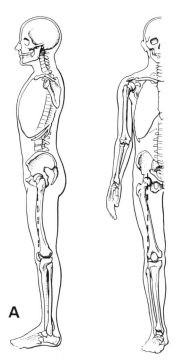

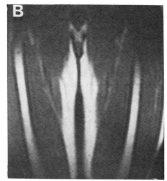

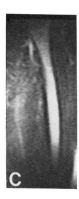

A

FIG. 13. Illustration of the angles of the extremities and spine in the coronal and sagittal planes (**A**). Coronal (**B**) and sagittal (**C**) images of the femurs demonstrating the partial volume effect (entire femur not on the image) due to the varus position of the femur in the coronal plane and anterior bowing in the sagittal plane.

difficult to maintain. Many patients must be allowed to rest periodically in order to complete the examination. If the patient is small enough the oblique position with the hand adjacent to the shoulder (elbow flexed) is more easily tolerated (Fig. 16C). The shoulders and upper humeri are currently examined with the arms at the side in either the body or corset coil. This position is comfortable, but image quality is not as optimal as when a surface coil is used. Use of surface coils in this situation requires off-axis placement (Fig. 16A), which reduces the effectiveness of the coil (Fig. 17). Improvements in software should solve some positioning problems.

Positioning and coil choices will be discussed more completely in later chapters as they apply to specific clinical problems.

PULSE SEQUENCES

Previous chapters (J. Nixon and R. L. Ehman, *this volume*) have discussed basic principles of MR pulse sequences and tissue characterization. Use of different pulse sequences (IR, spin–echo, free induction decay, and partial saturation) and the many available TE and TR selections would, at first, seem very confusing. However, current experience indicates that in most situations selection of a T1- and T2-weighted sequence will provide the necessary diagnostic information (4,18).

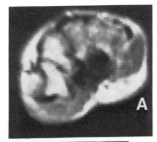
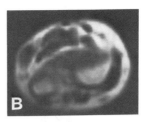
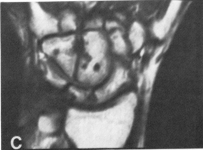

FIG. 14. Images of the wrist (**A**) and distal forearm (**B**) obtained using the same parameters (sequence and number of averages). The wrist was imaged in the head coil and the distal forearm in the small saddle (Fig. 8A) coil. **C:** 1.5 T surface coil image of the wrist showing multiple degenerative cysts in the carpal bones.

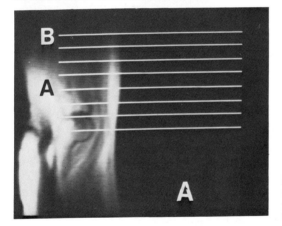
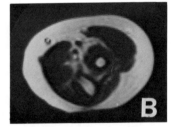
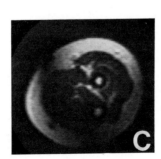
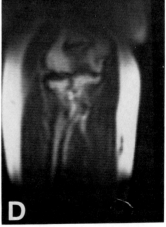

FIG. 15. Scout view of the proximal forearm and elbow for localization of an eight-section transaxial pulse sequence (TE 40, TR 133, time 19.5 sec). The transaxial image (**B**) taken near the center of the coil (A in Fig. 9A) is of excellent quality. The image obtained at the edge of the coil (**C**) is poor due to reduced signal. The margins of the coronal image (**D**) are also suboptimal.

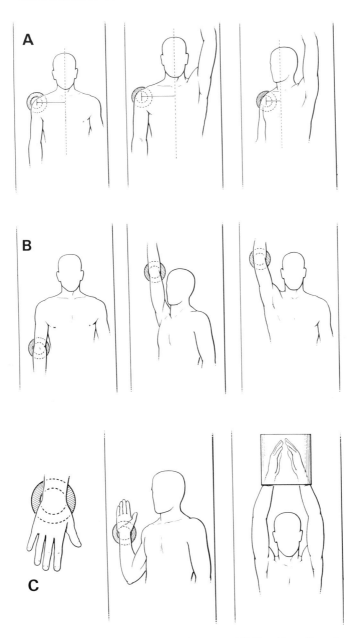

FIG. 16. Upper extremity positioning using surface coils. (**A**) Shoulder—the coil can be more easily centered by obliquing the patient and elevating the opposite extremity (**right**). (**B**) Elbow. (**C**) Wrists—hand at the side, **left;** elbow flexed, **middle;** both wrists above the head, **right.**

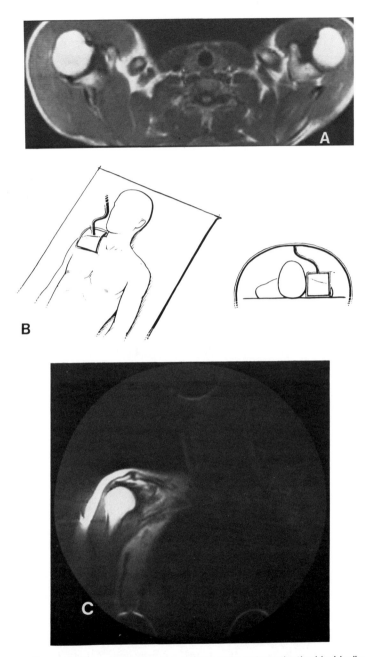

FIG. 17.   **A:** Transaxial view of the shoulders with the arms at the patient's side. Ideally a surface coil placed over the shoulder (**B**) would provide the best image. However, the coil and cable (insert in **B**) would be off-center and, therefore, the image (**C**) quality is reduced. Note that the volume of tissue imaged is also restricted. (See Fig. 15.)

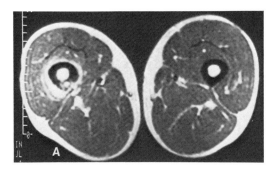

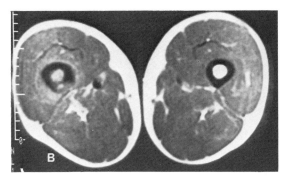

FIG. 18. Transaxial images of the thigh in a patient with lymphoma. The T2-weighted spin–echo image (TE 60, TR 2,000) (**A**) clearly shows the cortical and soft tissue involvement. The medullary involvement would be difficult to detect without the T1-weighted inversion recovery (TI 500, TR 1,500) image (**B**). Note that the degree of soft tissue involvement is not as well appreciated in **B**.

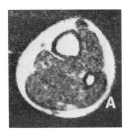 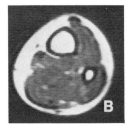

FIG. 19. Transaxial images of the lower leg using TE 30, TR 150. **A:** 1 average, time: 19 sec. **B:** 8 averages, time: 2 min, 34 sec.

Partial saturation (TE ≤ 25 and TR ≤ 500) and IR sequences are T1-weighted. Partial saturation sequences provide excellent image quality and can be performed quickly due to the short TR. The TR (150 to 500 msec) allows these sequences to be performed more than four times as fast as most IR sequences. The TRs commonly used with IR are in the 1,500 to 2,100 msec range. Abnormal tissues and fluid collections (long T1) appear dark using T1-weighted sequences. Therefore, they provide excellent contrast differentiation between normal marrow and fat (Fig. 18). Spin–echo sequences with long TE and TR (TE ≥ 60, TR ≥ 2000) are T2-weighted. Abnormal tissue (long T2) will have increased signal intensity allowing differentiation from muscle tissue, cortical bone, and fibrous structures (ligaments, tendon, scar tissue). Separation of abnormal tissue from fat or marrow may be difficult for fat has high signal intensity on both T1- and T2-weighted sequences (Fig. 18). Chemical shift imaging may be very useful in differentiating signal due to fat or water secondary to inflammation (19).

Image quality depends on many factors. We have already mentioned the importance of using the smallest coil possible. The signal-to-noise ratio may also be improved by increasing the number of averages (7) (Fig. 19). This increases scan time significantly [scan time = TR × number of averages × number of projections (128 or 256)]. Therefore, one must determine which factor is more important. The ultimate goal should be to obtain optimal image quality and information in the most reasonable amount of time.

With the clinical indication in mind, a thorough screening examination can usually be performed rather quickly. A scout image can be obtained in the coronal, sagittal, or axial plane using a partial saturation sequence with a TR of 150 msec. This image (Fig. 15) only takes 20 sec. Transaxial T2-weighted images can be performed using multisection multiecho sequences (Fig. 15) in 17 min or less. A T1-weighted partial saturation sequence can be performed in the coronal or sagittal plane in 4.5 min. Therefore, the total examination time is just under 22 min. Occasionally, more selected sequences may be required (IR, calculated T1 and T2 images, chemical shift, etc.). Advances in software will continue to add versatility and reduce examination time.

REFERENCES

1. Arakawa, M., Crooks, L. E., McCarten, B., Hoenninger, J. C., Watts, J. C., and Kaufman, L. (1985): A comparison of saddle shaped and solenoidal coils for magnetic resonance imaging. *Radiology,* 154:227–228.
2. Berquist, T. H. (1984): Preliminary experience in orthopedic radiology. *Magnetic Resonance Imaging,* 2:41–52.
3. Davis, P. L., Crooks, L., Arakawa, M., McRee, R., Kaufman, L., and Margulis, A. R. (1981): Potential hazards of MR imaging: Heating and effects of changing magnetic fields and RF fields on small metallic implants. *A. J. R.,* 137:857–860.
4. des Plantes, B. G. Z., Falke, T. H. M., and den Boer, J. A. (1984): Pulse sequences and contrast in magnetic resonance imaging. *Radiographics,* 4:869–883.
5. Fisher, M. R., Barker, B., Amparo, E. G., Brandt, G., Brant-Zawadzki, M., Hricak, H., and Higgins, C. B. (1985): MR imaging using specialized coils. *Radiology,* 157:443–447.

6. King, C. L., Henkelman, R. M., Poon, P. Y., and Rubenstein, J. (1984): MR imaging of the normal knee. *J. Comput. Assist. Tomogr.,* 8:1147–1154.
7. Kneeland, J. B., Knowles, R. J. R., and Cahill, P. T. (1984): Magnetic resonance imaging systems: Optimization in clinical use. *Radiology,* 153:473–478.
8. Lackman, R. W., Kaufman, B., Han, J. S., Nelson, D. A., Clampitt, M., O'Block, A. M., Haaga, J. R., and Alfidi, R. J. (1985): MR imaging in patients with metallic implants. *Radiology,* 157: 711–714.
9. Mechlin, M., Thickman, D., Kressel, H. Y., Gefter, W., and Joseph, P. (1984): Magnetic resonance imaging of postoperative patients with metallic implants. *A. J. R.,* 143:1281–1284.
10. Moon, K. L., Genant, H. K., Helms, C. A., Chafetz, N. I., Crooks, L. E., and Kaufman, L. (1983): Musculoskeletal applications of nuclear magnetic resonance. *Radiology,* 147:161–171.
11. New, P. F., Rosen, B. R., Brady, T. J., Buonanno, F., Kistler, J. P., Burt, C. T., Hinshaw, W. S., Newhouse, J. H., Pohost, G. M., and Taveras, J. M. (1983): Potential hazards and artifacts of ferromagnetic and nonferromagnetic surgical and dental materials and devices in nuclear magnetic resonance imaging. *Radiology,* 147:137–148.
12. Pavilcek, W., Geisinger, M., Castle, L., Barkowski, G. P., Meaney, T. F., Brean, B. L., and Gallagher, J. H. (1983): The effects of nuclear magnetic resonance on patients with cardiac pacemakers. *Radiology,* 147:149–153.
13. Roth, K. L., Nugent, M., Gray, J. E., Julsrud, P. R., Berquist, T. H., Sill, J. C., Kispert, D. B., and Hayes, D. L. (1985): Patient monitoring during magnetic resonance imaging. *Anesthesiology,* 62:80–83.
14. Saunders, R. D. (1982): Biological effects of NMR clinical imaging. *Appl. Radiol.,* 11:43–46.
15. Schenck, J. R., Hart, H. R., Foster, T. H., Edelstein, W. A., Bottomley, P. A., Redington, R. W., Hardy, C. J., Zimmerman, R. A., and Bilaniak, L. T. (1985): High field surface coil magnetic resonance imaging of localized anatomy. *Am. J. Neuroradiol.,* 6:193–196.
16. Schwartz, J. L., and Crooks, L. E. (1982): NMR imaging produces no observable mutations or cytotoxicity in mammalian cells. *A. J. R.,* 139:583–585.
17. Soulen, R. L., Budinger, T. F., and Higgins, C. B. (1985): Magnetic resonance imaging of prosthetic heart valves. *Radiology,* 154:705–707.
18. Wehrli, F. W., McFall, J. R., Glover, G. H., Grigsby, N., Haughton, V., and Johanson, J. (1984): The dependency of nuclear magnetic resonance image contrast on intrinsic and pulse sequence timing parameters. *Magnetic Resonance Imaging,* 2:3–16.
19. Wismer, G. L., Rosen, B. R., Buxton, R., Stark, D. B., and Brady, T. J. (1985): Chemical shift imaging of bone marrow: Preliminary experience. *A. J. R.,* 145:1031–1037.

Bone and Soft Tissue Tumors

Thomas H. Berquist

*Mayo Medical School, and Department of Diagnostic Radiology,
Mayo Clinic, Rochester, Minnesota 55905*

Limb salvage procedures generally provide the best functional result in management of bone and soft tissue tumors. It is important to have as much information as possible about the lesion to assess the chances of a surgical salvage procedure or to plan radiotherapy (23). The degree of neurovascular involvement, the extent of the lesion in bone and soft tissues, and the presence of skip lesions must be known (12,30). Physical examination and history may provide a presumptive diagnosis, but imaging techniques must be used to more clearly define the nature and extent of the lesions.

Routine radiographs and conventional tomograms are useful to evaluate and characterize skeletal lesions, but provide less information about soft tissue involvement. Xeroradiography has been used to evaluate lipomas and certain other soft tissue lesions. Ultrasound provides information about the texture, cystic or solid, of superficial lesions (1,9). Radionuclide scans, while useful for identification of lesions, have poor spatial resolution and may be inaccurate in determining the extent of lesions, in defining tumor margins, and in detecting skip lesions (5).

Until recently, computed tomography (CT) was the technique of choice in planning treatment of bone and soft tissue neoplasms (9,11,14,15,20,22,27). Recent studies have demonstrated that magnetic resonance (MR) imaging has certain advantages over CT and other imaging techniques which allow tumors to be more easily detected and their extent more clearly defined. The major advantages include: (a) direct coronal, sagittal, and transaxial imaging, (b) superior soft tissue contrast, (c) no beam hardening artifact from cortical bone, and (d) the ability to image patients with nonferromagnetic metal implants (2,10,17,18,26,30).

IMAGING TECHNIQUES

Imaging techniques and patient selection have been thoroughly discussed in previous chapters (R. L. Ehman and T. H. Berquist, "Technical Considerations in Magnetic Resonance Imaging," *this volume*). However, certain points need to be reemphasized. Identification of musculoskeletal neoplasms requires both T1 [partial saturation or inversion recovery (IR)] and T2 [spin–echo with echo time (TE) ≥ 60 and repetition time (TR) $\geq 2,000$ msec] weighted sequences to help differentiate true lesions from fatty replacement or lipomas. The T1-weighted sequences provide good fat–tumor contrast in the medullary canal and in soft tissues (Fig. 14). The T2-weighted sequences are best for detecting abnormalities in muscle and in cortical bone, but less effective in medullary bone and in areas of adipose tissue where fat–tumor contrast is reduced unless very long TR is used. Fat maintains a high signal intensity on most commonly used pulse sequences (Fig. 3). In certain cases, spin–echo sequences with longer TE (≥ 80) and TR ($\geq 3,000$) may be useful to detect subtle abnormalities in fatty tissue or to differentiate tumor from edema (tumor signal intensity is less than edema). Sequences with long TR are not commonly used because the examination time is significantly increased.

The extent of a lesion is best assessed with coronal or sagittal images used in combination with transaxial images. Coronal images have the additional advantage of allowing comparison of both extremities. It is not usually necessary to perform both T1- and T2-weighted sequences in more than one plane unless subtraction (see R. L. Ehman, *this volume*) is needed. Generally, a T1-weighted sequence can be performed in the coronal or sagittal plane and a T2-weighted sequence in the transaxial plane. This reduces examination time and improves patient throughput.

The patient should be positioned so that soft tissues in the area of interest are not distorted. For example, if the suspected pathology is in the calf, the patient should be prone. The smallest, most closely coupled coil available should be used to maximize image quality, providing that it has a sufficiently large field of view.

PRIMARY BONE AND SOFT TISSUE TUMORS

The value of magnetic resonance (MR) imaging in studies of musculoskeletal neoplasms is becoming more evident in clinical practice and the scientific literature. Over 175 cases have been reported in the literature (2–6,21,26,29–31). At our institution, we have studied over 300 patients with malignant and benign primary tumors, metastasis, or suspected local recurrence.

Primary Bone Tumors

Routine radiographs provide valuable information for determining the benign or malignant nature of bone lesions (8). MR imaging is most commonly used to further evaluate lesions which are either equivocal or obviously malignant. MR imaging also provides more information about the extent of bone and soft tissue involvement and also allows detection of subtle lesions which may be overlooked on radiographs.

Previously, computed tomography (CT) was considered the "gold standard" for planning treatment of bone tumors (12,14,20). This may now be changing. MR imaging has better soft tissue resolution than CT which allows lesions to be more easily detected. Also, the lack of beam-hardening artifact from cortical bone results in better assessment of juxtacortical tissues (10). Detection of skip lesions and the extent of medullary bone involvement is more readily accomplished with MR imaging than CT (Fig. 1). It has been reported that MR imaging is superior to CT in assessing medullary involvement in 33% of cases. Soft tissue extent was more readily appreciated in 38% of cases. CT, however, was superior in detection of subtle calcifications, which may appear as small areas of reduced signal intensity on MR images or they may not be seen at all. Pathologic fractures were also more easily seen with CT (30). However, with improvements in software and surface coils these advantages may not persist.

Primary Soft Tissue Tumors

As with bone tumors, CT has been the technique of choice for evaluation of soft tissue masses (9,10,14,20,27). In a recent review of 84 patients with untreated

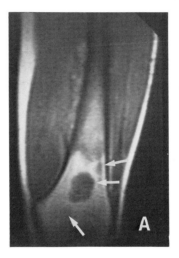
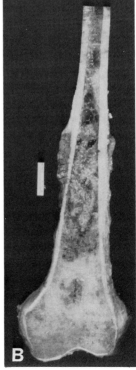

FIG. 1. Patient with Grade IV osteosarcoma. **A:** Coronal MR image (TE 40, TR 500) shows the main lesion plus several skip lesions (*arrows*) distally. **B:** The pathologic specimen closely matches the MR image. (From Zimmer et al., ref. 30, with permission.)

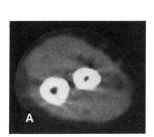
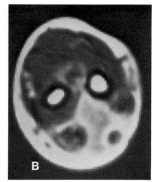
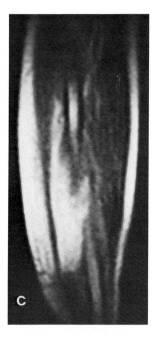

FIG. 2. Recurrent desmoid tumor in the forearm. **A:** CT scan is difficult to interpret without the opposite extremity for comparison. The mass is the same density as muscle. Axial (**B**) and coronal (**C**) MR images (TE 60, TR 2,000) clearly identify the lesion (high signal intensity) and the degree of involvement.

soft tissue neoplasms, CT demonstrated the lesion in each case and provided adequate anatomic definition in the majority of patients (27). Histology was often difficult to predict from CT images, but in 88% of patients, the authors were able to differentiate benign from malignant lesions. CT was not as effective in the neck, shoulder, and peripheral extremities (27).

Recent studies, including our experience in over 150 patients, indicate that MR imaging is generally superior to CT in lesion detection and characterizing the extent of involvement of adjacent bone and soft tissue structures (10,26,30). With CT, the density of a soft tissue mass is often similar to muscle, necessitating careful comparison with the opposite extremity and changes in window widths and levels to identify the lesion. Lesion detection is especially difficult in the peripheral extremities where muscle planes are not as clearly defined by surrounding adipose tissue (Fig. 2). Weekes et al. (26) reviewed CT and MR imaging findings in 27 patients with soft tissue tumors. In all but one case, MR imaging was better or at least equal to CT in defining the anatomic extent of the lesion. The increased soft tissue contrast, as well as the coronal and sagittal imaging capability of MR imaging, were largely responsible for the added information. This was particularly true in the distal extremities. MR imaging was also superior in demonstrating neurovascular involvement, without use of contrast material to visualize vessels.

CHARACTERIZATION OF TUMORS

Evaluation of the imaging features, tissue characterization, and specificity of MR imaging is still in progress. It has been clearly demonstrated that T1 and

TABLE 1. *Relaxation times (msec)*

	T1	T2
Malignant tumors	400–887	195–278
Benign tumors	375–628	132–246
Infection	572–613	404–433
Cysts	700–800	400–500
Hematoma	376–559	146–282

T2 relaxation times are prolonged in neoplastic tissue (19,30,31). It was hoped that calculation of relaxation times using routine imaging sequences would provide additional data which, along with image characteristics, could increase the diagnostic specificity. The accuracy of these calculations has been questioned. However, phantom studies have indicated that T1 and T2 values can be consistently reproduced on a given unit providing that care is taken with the technique (13). The relaxation time values will vary with field strength and other technical details which are specific to different imagers. Data that has been generated thus far indicates that there is considerable overlap of relaxation times making current calculations less useful in predicting tumor histology and in differentiating tumors from other pathology (7,23–25,30,31) (Table 1).

Image characteristics, on the other hand, are useful for predicting the nature of lesions. Certain criteria, such as morphology, can be applied to MR images in the same way that they are to CT and radiography.

Most benign musculoskeletal tumors that are imaged with MR imaging at our institution are soft tissue neoplasms as benign bone lesions can usually be well characterized with routine radiographs. With the exception of desmoids,

TABLE 2. *MR features: soft tissue tumors*

	Benign	Malignant
Margins Irregular or hazy	Uncommon	Common
Texture	Homogeneous	Inhomogeneous
Signal intensity T2 (TE 60, TR 2000+)	High (white)	Intermediate (>muscle) mixed white and dark
T1 (IR-T1 500, TE 40, TR 1,500–2,000)	Low (black)[a]	Intermediate (>muscle) mixed white and dark
Partial saturation (TE 25, TR ≤ 500)	≥Muscle	≤Muscle, mixed intensity
Neurovascular involvement	Rare	Common
Bone involvement	None	Uncommon

[a] Lipomas are high intensity on all of the above sequences.

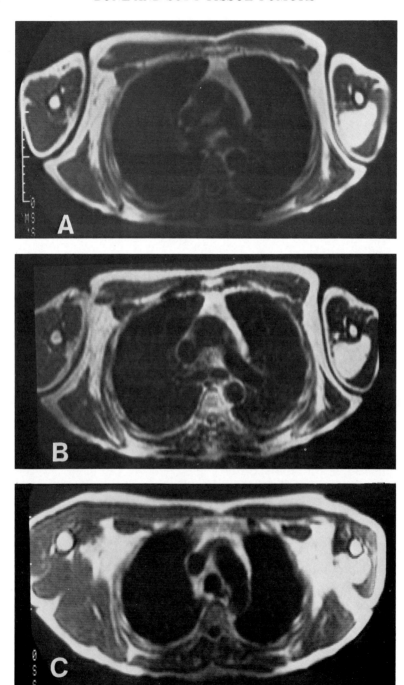

FIG. 3. Benign lipoma. There is a well marginated high signal intensity lesion similar to fat in the upper humerus. The lesion maintains the same appearance on partial saturation (**A**), IR (TI 500, TE 40, TR 1,500) (**B**), and spin–echo (TE 60, TR 200) (**C**) sequences.

hemangiomas, and arteriovenous malformations, benign soft tissue tumors have fairly characteristic features (Table 2). They are homogeneous and well margin-ated; the signal intensity is increased (white) on T2-weighted sequences and decreased (dark or black) on T1-weighted images. Lipomas are of high intensity on T1- and T2-weighted sequences (Fig. 3). Bone and neurovascular involvement is rare.

There is now sufficient experience with certain types of tumors to describe their specific MR features.

Lipomas

As with CT, lipomas have the most constant MR appearance (9,26,27) and maintain a high signal intensity in T1- and T2-weighted sequences. They are well marginated with occasional thin fibrous septations, but they are generally not as inhomogeneous as liposarcomas. Liposarcomas and other malignant le-sions can usually be differentiated by their mixed density, irregular margins, and decreased signal intensity on T1-weighted images. Neurovascular structures are also commonly involved (Fig. 4).

Cysts

Bone and soft tissue cysts are well marginated and usually have a well defined capsule. The signal intensity varies with the type of fluid, but is usually high (white) on T2-weighted and low (black) on T1-weighted sequences. Complicated or hemorrhagic cysts have an intermediate signal intensity (Figs. 5 and 6).

Fibromas

Fibromas are intermediate in intensity on both T1- and T2-weighted sequences. Most are small and well defined (Fig. 7). The exceptions are mixed tumors such

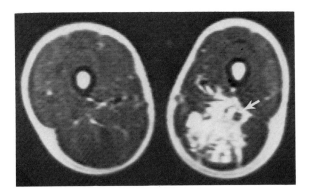

FIG. 4. Axial image (TE 60, TR 2,000) through the thigh in a patient with a liposarcoma. Note the mixed signal intensity, vascular involvement (*arrow*), and irregular margins.

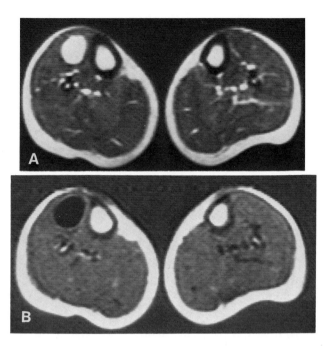

FIG. 5. Benign simple cyst near the upper tibia. **A:** T2-weighted image (TE 60, TR 2,000) shows a uniform high-intensity lesion with a thin low-intensity capsule. **B:** IR (TI 500, TE 40, TR 1,500) demonstrates a uniformly dark lesion due to long T1.

as neurofibromas which may be large and difficult to differentiate from malignant lesions (high intensity on T2- and low intensity on T1-weighted sequences).

Hemangiomas

Unlike most benign lesions, hemangiomas and arteriovenous malformations are often irregular, mixed density, due to numerous vessels, and diffuse or multiple. Large serpiginous vessels are often present, but identification of feeding vessels or specific arteries and veins is usually not possible (Figs. 8 and 9). Clinical history and the presence of numerous vessels almost always allow differentiation from malignant lesions.

Desmoids

Desmoid tumors are locally aggressive infiltrating fibrous lesions that tend to recur following resection. They are most common in the third and fifth decades and do not metastasize (8,16). The most common location (11/25 patients) was in the shoulder, with calf, forearm, and buttock each involved in 4 patients. The

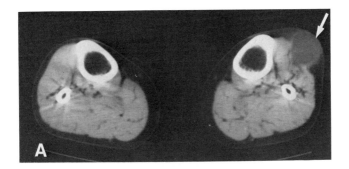

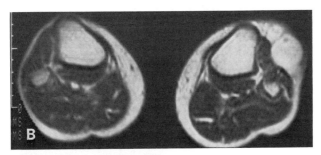

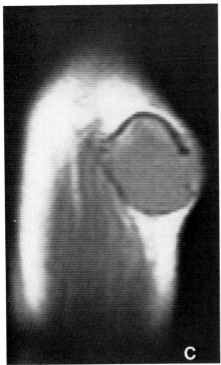

FIG. 6. Ganglion cyst near the knee. **A:** CT scan demonstrates an intermediate density lesion with a thick capsule (*arrow*). **B:** Axial MR image (TE 60, TR 2,000) reveals a uniform high signal intensity lesion which is intermediate in density on the partial saturation (**C**) sagittal image.

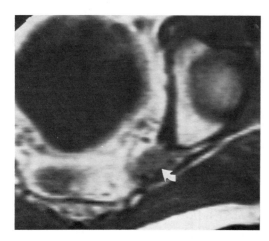

FIG. 7. Benign fibroma (*arrow*) near the sciatic nerve (TE 60, TR 2,000). The density is only slightly higher than muscle on this sequence.

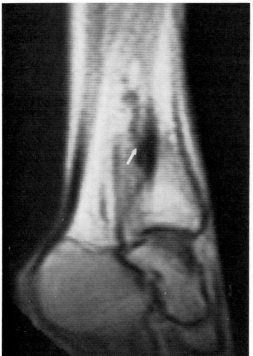

FIG. 8. Arteriovenous malformation of the ankle with the serpiginous vessels (*arrow*) clearly seen on the partial saturation sagittal MR image.

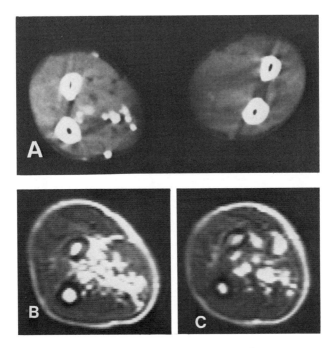

FIG. 9. Hemangioma of the forearm. **A:** CT scan with contrast shows numerous contrast filled vessels in the forearm. Axial MR images (**B, C**) demonstrate an irregular high intensity lesion with multiple vessels. (Signal can be noted in vessels on multislice images as in this eight-section TE 60, TR 2,000 sequence.)

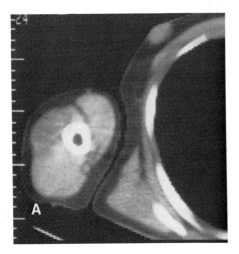
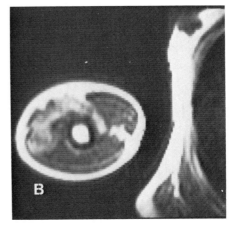

FIG. 10. Desmoid tumor of the upper arm. **A:** CT scan shows a subtle area of decreased density in the muscles of the arm lateral to the humerus. Note the streaking due to beam hardening artifact from cortical bone. **B:** Axial MR image (TE 60, TR 2,000) performed in a closely coupled extremity coil shows a high signal intensity lesion with irregular margins extending around the anterior humerus.

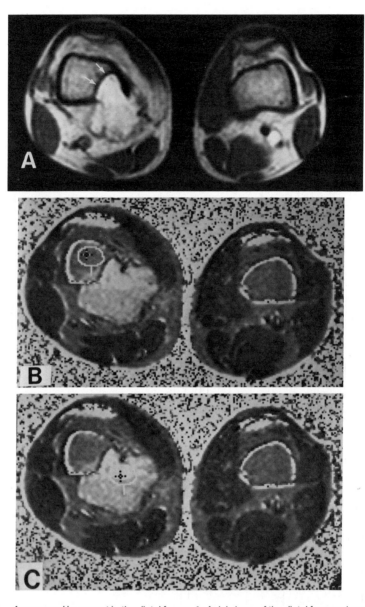

FIG. 11. Aneurysmal bone cyst in the distal femur. **A:** Axial views of the distal femurs demonstrate a high intensity lesion projecting from the right femur. The lesion is separated from normal medullary bone by a low intensity rim of fiber bone (*arrows*). T2 calculations of the normal marrow (**B**) and tumor (**C**) were 81 and 205 msec, respectively.

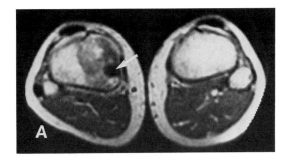

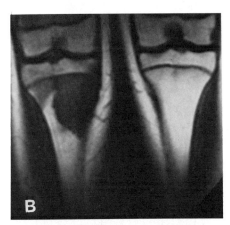

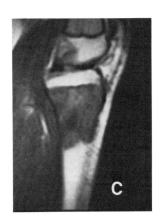

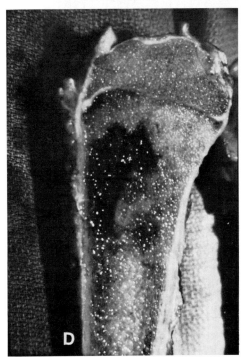

FIG. 12. Osteoblastic osteosarcoma of the proximal tibia. **A:** Axial view (TE 40, TR 2,000) shows a mixed density lesion with bone sclerosis (*arrow*). Coronal (**B**) and sagittal (**C**) images clearly demonstrate the extent of the lesion and correlate with the pathologic specimen (**D**). (From Zimmer et al., ref. 30, with permission.)

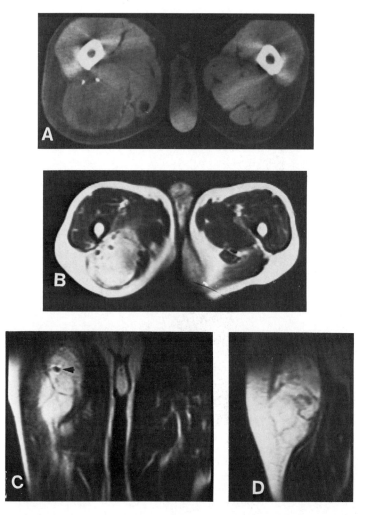

FIG. 13. Liposarcoma. **A:** CT scan shows a low density mass in the thigh with several surgical clips. **B:** Axial T2-weighted MR images show the mass with low density areas surrounded by halos due to surgical clip artifact. Vessels do not have the same appearance. Coronal (**C**) and sagittal (**D**) images demonstrate the clip artifact (*arrow*) with inhomogeneity of the tumor and encasement of vessels by the tumor.

MR appearance does not follow the pattern of typical benign lesions: in our recent review of 25 cases, we noted that 80% were inhomogeneous, and the margins were irregular or infiltrative in keeping with the pathology of the lesion (Fig. 10). The intensity of the lesions was slightly greater than muscle with short TE and TR (40/500), intermediate to high intensity on T2-weighted sequences, and slightly decreased intensity on T1-weighted sequences. MR imaging was superior to CT in detecting and determining the extent of the lesions.

MR experience in diagnosis of benign bone lesions is more limited, as routine radiographs are usually adequate to define and characterize the lesion. MR appearance varies depending on the type of tumor matrix (cartilage, fibrous, osteoid, etc.), but a clearly defined low-intensity margin was noted in 33% of our patients and in patients with osteomyelitis (30,31) (Fig. 11). Malignant lesions rarely have this appearance.

Malignant Tumors

Most malignant bone and soft tissue tumors are inhomogeneous with mixed signal intensity on both T1- and T2-weighted sequences (Table 2). This appearance may be secondary to tumor necrosis, calcification, or the type of tumor matrix (osteoid, fibrous, cartilaginous) (29,30) (Fig. 12). Areas of calcification or bone formation appear dark, like cortical bone, on all pulse sequences. These areas are usually irregular and easily differentiated from vessels. Surgical clips with ferromagnetic impurities may also cause dark artifacts, but they usually have a white halo due to local image distortion (Figs. 13 and 14). Some malignant tumors appear fairly well marginated. In these lesions, neurovascular engulfment may be the only indication of malignancy (Fig. 14). The latter feature and inhomogeneity are the most reliable MR imaging indicators of malignancy in soft tissue tumors.

Histologic differentiation of malignant lesions is difficult with current techniques. We have not found calculated T1 and T2 values or image appearance to be particularly helpful in this regard. Certain features may be useful occasionally. For example, lymphoma of bone tends to have a more uniform, low-intensity appearance in the medullary cavity on partial saturation sequences. This may be most easily appreciated on coronal or sagittal views (Fig. 15). On

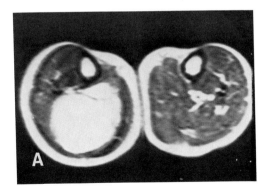
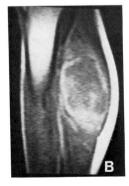

FIG. 14. Malignant fibrous histiocytoma. **A:** T2-weighted image (TE 60, TR 2,000) demonstrates a high intensity lesion slightly irregular margins. This could be confused with a lipoma if only one pulse sequence were used. **B:** Sagittal partial saturation image demonstrates the inhomogeneity and mixed signal intensity seen with malignant lesions.

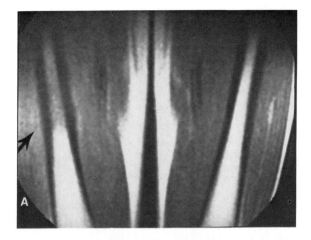

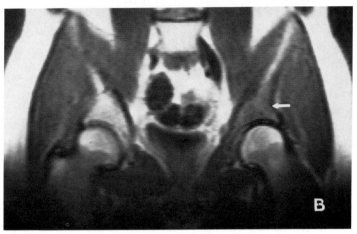

FIG. 15.   Lymphoma of bone. **A:** Coronal (TE 40, TR 500) images of the femurs demonstrate a uniform decrease in signal in the medullary bone (*arrow*) due to lymphoma. **B:** Coronal image of the pelvis with the same pulse sequence shows decreased intensity in the left innominate bone due to lymphoma.

T2-weighted sequences with a TE of 60 and TR of 2,000, the tumor is difficult to distinguish from normal marrow.

As previously mentioned, detection of subtle soft tissue calcification is often useful in classifying tumors (Fig. 16), and in this situation CT may be more useful. However, even if calcifications are evident on routine radiographs, MR is still the technique of choice to evaluate the extent of the lesion.

Differential Diagnosis

Certain conditions may be difficult to differentiate clinically and with imaging techniques from neoplasm.

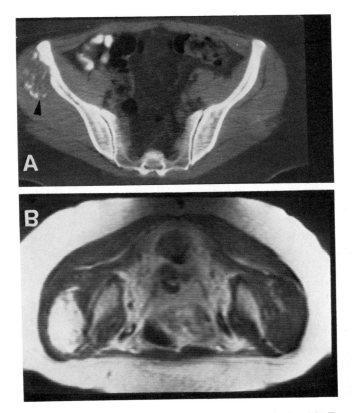

FIG. 16. Chondrosarcoma of the ilium. **A:** CT scan shows a lesion in the right ilium with soft tissue calcification (*arrow*). **B:** MR image (TE 60, TR 2,000) clearly demonstrates the soft tissue involvement. The calcium is seen as areas of no signal.

Soft tissue trauma may lead to intramuscular hemorrhage, hematoma, inflammation, and myositis ossificans. Differentiation of these lesions from soft tissue tumors with MR is not always possible, but certain imaging features are helpful. Inflammatory change and intraparenchymal hemorrhage have a similar feathery, infiltrative appearance (Fig. 17). The signal intensity is high on T2-weighted images and low on T1-weighted images, which also allows differentiation from fatty infiltration or atrophy which has a high intensity on both sequences. Hematomas tend to be well marginated and confined to the involved muscle or tissue space. The texture is homogeneous initially, but as the clot organizes, the lesion develops a mixed appearance due to the presence of fibrin clot, methemaglobin, and liquid plasma. The relaxation times of both hemorrhage and hematoma decrease over a period of 2 to 3 weeks, unlike the constant relaxation times of simple edema and tumors (24).

Diagnosis of myositis can be difficult with both MR and CT in the early inflammatory stages (9,20). Once ossified, the MR appearance would be similar to cortical bone.

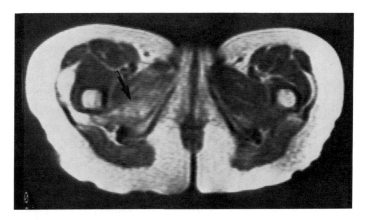

FIG. 17. Axial (TE 60, TR 2,000) image in a patient with nodular polymyositis involving the adductor muscles. Note the infiltrative pattern (*arrow*). Neoplasms are more localized and more clearly separated from normal tissue.

Soft tissue abscesses have certain features which may help distinguish them from tumors. Though experience is limited, abscesses we have studied have a thick irregular capsule which is uncommon with tumors and not like the thin walled capsule of a simple cyst (Fig. 18). Unlike CT, no contrast is required to define the capsule with MR imaging (7,25). The pattern of the contents is also more inhomogeneous than simple or complicated cysts.

Bone lesions such as fibrous dysplasia or Paget's disease can also mimic tumors. To date, MR experience with these lesions is too limited to develop differential diagnostic criteria.

Metastatic Disease

Metastases frequently involve the axial skeleton. Radionuclide scans have been very useful in detection of early metastasis, but certain lesions such as myeloma may be difficult to detect. Radiographic surveys are also commonly used, but subtle lesions can be easily overlooked.

The role of MR imaging in the evaluation of skeletal metastasis has not been established. However, potential exists, especially in the axial skeleton. The sensitivity of the technique has been clearly established (2,17,26–28), and detection of lesions not seen on radiographs or nuclear scans is possible. Differentiation of osteoporotic compression or degenerative wedging of vertebrae from metastases can be particularly troublesome. Tomography is of little value in these patients. MR images are useful in detecting the focal lesions of myeloma or metastasis (Fig. 19). Compressed osteoporotic vertebrae have uniform signal intensity. If metastasis or myeloma are present, the signal intensity will change (increased T2-weighted, decreased T1-weighted) compared to the uninvolved portion of the vertebra. Sagittal images of the spine can be quickly obtained, allowing eval-

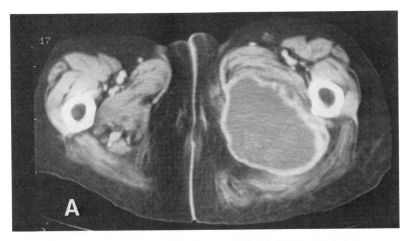

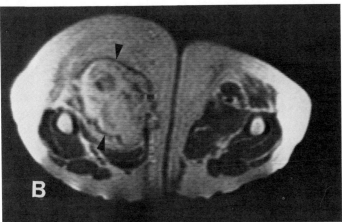

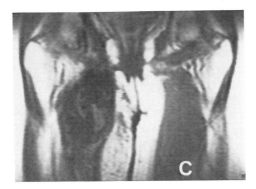

FIG. 18. Thigh abscess. **A:** CT scan with contrast demonstrates a large low density lesion with an enhancing capsule. **B:** Axial MR image (TE 60, TR 2,000) shows a mixed intensity lesion with a thick low intensity capsule (*arrows*). Coronal image (**C**) using partial saturation demonstrates a predominantly low intensity lesion which makes the capsule more difficult to identify.

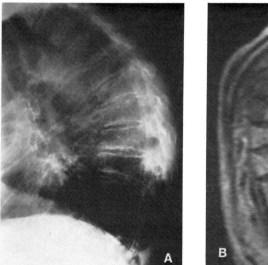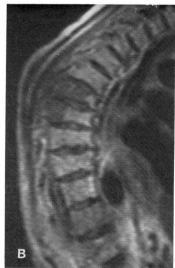

FIG. 19. Degenerative wedging and osteoporosis in a patient with suspected metastasis. **A:** Lateral radiograph of the thoracic spine shows these changes. It is difficult to be certain if there are underlying metastases. **B:** Sagittal MR image (TE 30, TR 500) shows focal areas of decreased signal in the areas involved with metastasis.

uation of the skeletal structures and spinal canal. In future, detection of obstructing lesions may obviate the need for myelography prior to radiation therapy or surgical decompression.

Currently, the time required to survey the entire skeleton is prohibitive. However, if suspicious extraaxial areas on radiographs or isotope scans are present, MR imaging is useful to confirm and characterize the abnormality. This is especially important if radiation therapy or surgery is considered.

Posttreatment Evaluation

Evaluation of patients with suspected tumor recurrence presents a difficult problem. Differentiation of postoperative changes from recurrence is difficult with most imaging modalities, especially in the early postoperative period. Hudson et al. (11) reviewed 21 patients with suspected recurrence of sarcomas and found that CT was unable to detect microscopic tumor. It was also difficult to differentiate recurrence from hematoma. In contrast, MR imaging has potential to separate recurrence from hemorrhage or postoperative changes, as indicated by Swensen in his study of hematoma evolution (24). In the later phases of healing, scar tissue has a lower signal intensity than normal tissue due to a lower mobile spin density and shorter T2. Sequences with long TR and TE parameters are useful for differentiating recurrent tumor from scar tissue. They may also be

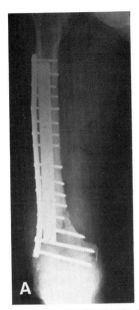

FIG. 20. Recurrent malignant fibrous histiocytoma of the femur. **A:** AP radiograph demonstrating double plate and screw fixation. **B:** The information on the CT scan is significantly reduced by metal artifact. **C:** MR image shows some artifact, but the tumor (high intensity) is clearly seen. (From Zimmer et al., ref. 30, with permission.)

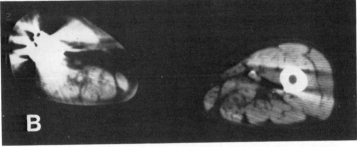

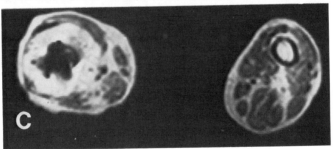

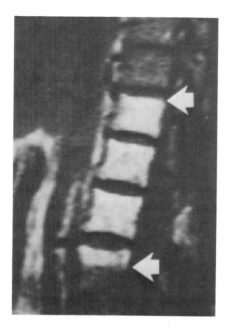

FIG. 21. Radiation changes in the lumbar spine. There is increased signal intensity, probably due to fatty replacement of marrow (*arrows*), in the region of the radiation port. (From Ramsey and Zacharias, ref. 18, with permission.)

helpful for distinguishing tumor from edema and inflammation changes as the latter tend to have a higher signal intensity. Much more work is needed to clarify the role of MR in this situation.

With the increase in the use of limb salvage procedures, patients frequently have metal implants, making CT evaluation of recurrence very difficult due to extensive artifact formation. We have found MR to be the technique of choice in this group of patients. The majority of orthopedic appliances (see T. H. Berquist, "Technical Considerations in Magnetic Resonance Imaging," *this volume*) are nonferromagnetic, causing little artifact in MR images. Recurrence or lack of recurrence can be more easily established with MR imaging (2,28) (Fig. 20).

Differentiation of recurrent tumor from radiation changes can also be difficult. Ramsey and Zacharias (18) described the MR changes in the spine following radiation therapy (Fig. 21). On T1-weighted images (TE 30, TR 500) the signal intensity of the irradiated vertebrae was increased, whereas pathologic tissue usually has a lower intensity. The increased signal intensity is believed to be due to fatty replacement. We have noted similar changes in soft tissues following radiation therapy.

SUMMARY

Routine radiographs remain effective in characterizing many skeletal lesions. Radionuclide scans are especially useful in detecting skeletal metastasis (14). CT

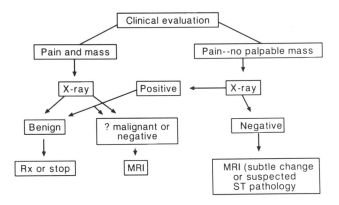

FIG. 22. Algorithm demonstrating the use of MR imaging in primary bone and soft tissue tumors.

is a valuable tool for evaluating tumors of the musculoskeletal system, and it is especially efficacious in identifying pulmonary metastases. The impact of MR imaging is still being evaluated. Tissue specificity and spectroscopy in the musculoskeletal system are in early stages of evaluation (28), but even in the development stage, advantages over current techniques in evaluation of bone and soft tissue tumors are evident. MR is superior to CT in evaluation of medullary bone, joint, and soft tissue involvement in many patients with musculoskeletal tumors (Fig. 22). The use of MR imaging in patients with nonferromagnetic metallic implants is also advantageous. CT is effective for detecting subtle calcifications and pathologic fractures. The effectiveness of MR imaging in this regard has improved significantly with the development of newer software and surface coils.

REFERENCES

1. Bernardino, M. E., Jing, B. S., Thomas, J. L., Lindell, M. M., Jr., and Zornoza, J. (1981): The extremity soft tissue lesion: A comparison of ultrasound, computed tomography, and xeroradiography. *Diagn. Radiol.,* 139:53–59.
2. Berquist, T. H. (1984): Magnetic resonance imaging: Preliminary experience in orthopedic radiology. *Magnetic Resonance Imaging,* 2:41–52.
3. Brady, T. J., Gebhardt, M. C., Pykett, I. L., Buonnano, F. S., Newhouse, J. H., Burt, C. T., Smith, R. J., Mankin, H. J., Kistler, J. P., Goldman, M. R., Hinshaw, W. S., and Pohost, G. M. (1982): NMR imaging of the forearms in healthy volunteers and patients with giant cell tumors of bone. *Radiology,* 144:549–552.
4. Brady, T. J., Rosen, B. R., Pykett, I. L., McGuire, M. H., Mankin, H. J., and Rosenthal, D. I. (1983): NMR imaging of leg tumors. *Radiology,* 149:181–187.
5. Chew, F. S., and Hudson, T. M. (1982): Radionuclear bone scanning of osteosarcoma: Falsely extended patterns of uptake. *A. J. R.,* 139:49–54.
6. Cohen, M. D., Klatte, E. C., Baehner, R., Smith, J. A., Mortin-Simmerman, P., Carr, B. E., Provisor, A. T., Weetman, B. M., Coates, T., Siddiqui, A., Weisman, S. J., Berkow, R., McKenna, S., and McGuire, W. A. (1984): Magnetic resonance imaging of bone marrow disease in children. *Radiology,* 151:715–718.
7. Cohen, J. M., Weinreb, J. C., and Maravilla, K. R. (1985): Fluid collections in the intraperitoneal and extraperitoneal spaces: Comparison of MR and CT. *Radiology,* 155:705–708.

8. Dahlin, D. (1978): *Bone Tumors: General Aspects and Data on 6,211 Cases.* Charles C. Thomas, Springfield, Illinois.

9. Heiken, J. P., Lee, L. K. T., Smathers, R. L., Toffy, W. G., and Murphy, W. A. (1984): CT of benign soft tissue masses of the extremities. *A. J. R.,* 142:575–580.

10. Hudson, T. M., Hamlin, D. J., Enneking, W. F., and Petterson, H. (1985): Magnetic resonance imaging of bone and soft tissue tumors: Early experience in 31 patients compared to computed tomography. *Skeletal Radiol.,* 13:134–146.

11. Hudson, T. M., Schakel, M., II, and Springfield, D. S. (1985): Limitations of computed tomography following excisional biopsy of soft tissue sarcomas. *Skeletal Radiol.,* 13:49–54.

12. Hudson, T. M., Schiebler, M., Springfield, D. S., Hawkins, I. R., Jr., Enneking, W. F., and Spanier, S. S. (1983): Radiologic imaging of osteosarcoma: Role in planning surgical treatment. *Skeletal Radiol.,* 10:137–146.

13. Kjos, B. O., Ehman, R. L., and Brant-Zawadzski, M. (1985): Reproducibility of T1 and T2 relaxation times calculated from routine MR imaging sequences: Phantom study. *A. J. R.,* 144: 1157–1163.

14. Levine, E., Lee, K. R., Neff, J. R., Maklad, N. F., Robinson, R. G., and Preston, D. F. (1979): Comparison of computed tomography and other image modalities in evaluation of musculoskeletal tumors. *Radiology,* 131:431–437.

15. Lukens, J. A., McLeod, R. A., and Sim, F. H. (1982): Computed tomography of primary osseous neurologic neoplasms. *A. J. R.,* 139:45–48.

16. McDougall, A., and McGarrity, G. (1979): Extra-abdominal desmoid tumors. *J. Bone Joint Surg.* [*Br.*], 61:373–377.

17. Moon, K. L., Genant, H. K., Helms, C. A., Chafetz, N. I., Crooks, L. E., and Kaufman, L. (1983): Musculoskeletal applications of nuclear magnetic resonance. *Radiology,* 147:161–171.

18. Ramsey, R. G., and Zacharias, C. E. (1985): MR imaging of the spine after radiation therapy: Easily recognizable effects. *A. J. R.,* 144:1131–1135.

19. Ranade, S. S., Shah, S. H., Advani, S. H., and Kasturi, S. R. (1977): Pulsed nuclear magnetic resonance studies in human bone marrow. *Physiol. Chem. Phys.,* 9:297–299.

20. Rosenthal, D. I. (1982): Computed tomography in bone and soft tissue neoplasm: Application and pathologic correlation. *C. R. C. Crit. Rev. Diagn. Imag.,* 18:243–277.

21. Rosenthal, D. I., Scott, J. A., Mankin, H. J., Wismer, G. L., and Brady, T. J. (1985): Saccrococcygeal chordoma. Magnetic resonance imaging and computed tomography. *A. J. R.,* 145:143–147.

22. Scott, J. A., Rosenthal, D. I., and Brady, T. J. (1984): The evaluation of musculoskeletal disease with magnetic resonance imaging. *Radiol. Clin. North Am.,* 22:917–924.

23. Shuman, W. P., Griffin, B. R., Haymor, D. R., Johnson, J. S., Jones, D. C., Cromwell, L. D., and Moss, A. A. (1985): MR imaging in radiation therapy planning. *Radiology,* 156:143–147.

24. Swensen, S. T., Keller, P. L., Berquist, T. H., McLeod, R. A., and Stephens, D. H. (1985): Magnetic resonance of hemorrhage. *A. J. R.,* 145:921–927.

25. Wall, S. D., Fisher, M. R., Amporo, E. G., Hricak, H., and Higgins, C. B. (1985): Magnetic resonance imaging in evaluation of abscesses. *A. J. R.,* 144:1217–1221.

26. Weekes, R. G., Berquist, T. H., McLeod, R. A., and Zimmer, W. D. (1985): Magnetic resonance imaging of soft tissue tumors: Comparison with CT. *Magnetic Resonance Imaging,* 3(4):345–352.

27. Weekes, R. G., McLeod, R. A., Reiman, H. M., and Pritchard, D. J. (1985): CT of soft tissue neoplasms. *A. J. R.,* 144:355–360.

28. Wismer, G. L., Rosen, B. R., Buxton, R., Stark, D. D., and Brady, T. J. (1985): Chemical shift imaging of bone marrow: Preliminary experience. *A. J. R.,* 145:1031–1037.

29. Zimmer, W. D., Berquist, T. H., McLeod, R. A., Pritchard, D. J., Shives, T. C., Wold, L. E., and May, G. R. (1986): MRI of osteosarcoma. *Clin. Orthop. (in press).*

30. Zimmer, W. D., Berquist, T. H., McLeod, R. A., Sim, F. H., Pritchard, D. J., Shives, T. C., Wold, L. E., and May, G. R. (1985): Magnetic resonance imaging of bone tumors: Comparison with CT. *Radiology,* 155:709–718.

31. Zimmer, W. D., Berquist, T. H., Sim, F. H., Pritchard, D. J., Shives, T. C., Wold, L. E., and May, G. R. (1985): Magnetic resonance imaging of aneurysmal bone cyst. *Mayo Clin. Proc.,* 59: 633–666.

Musculoskeletal Infection

Thomas H. Berquist

Mayo Medical School, and Department of Diagnostic Radiology,
Mayo Clinic, Rochester, Minnesota 55905

Musculoskeletal infections may present with an acute, rapidly progressing course or in a more insidious fashion. The latter often follow trauma or surgery, such as after placement of orthopedic appliances (7). Early treatment, particularly in children with articular infections, is essential to prevent growth defects or joint ankylosis (11). Determination of the extent of involvement is important in planning proper medical or surgical management. Routine radiographs and computed tomography (CT) are useful for this purpose. Radioisotope studies are particularly sensitive in the early stages of infection (5,7,11,18).

Skeletal infections typically begin in medullary bone. The resulting hyperemia and inflammation cause alterations in the intensity of medullary bone on magnetic resonance (MR) images (4,11,18). The excellent tissue contrast and multiplanar imaging provided by MR imaging may allow earlier and more accurate assessment than current imaging techniques (3,4,17,19). Therefore, acute osteomyelitis may be evident on MR images when radiographs and CT are negative (4,11).

Discussion of the utility of MR imaging is facilitated by categorizing patients in the following manner: (a) infection in nonviolated tissue, (b) infection in violated tissue (previous trauma or surgery), and (c) evaluation of surgical techniques for treatment. The latter category includes patients treated with muscle or omental flaps and vascularized fibular grafts.

INFECTION IN NONVIOLATED TISSUE

Osteomyelitis presents a diagnostic and therapeutic challenge regardless of the age group. Early diagnosis and management are essential to avoid irreversible bone and soft tissue damage. Hematogenous osteomyelitis, which occurs more commonly in children than adults, may be acute, subacute, or chronic, and most commonly involves the long bones of the lower extremities. In neonates and adults, the epiphysis is not protected: vascular channels cross the growth plate allowing infection to involve both the metaphysis and epiphysis with a high incidence of joint space involvement (5,7,22). In patients 1 to 16 years of age, the growth plate prevents spread of infection to the epiphyses, and joint space involvement is less common unless the metaphysis is intracapsular (5).

Infections typically involve the metaphyseal portion of long bones or areas near the physis in flat bones, such as the ilium. Radiologic changes are nonspecific in the early stages of infection. Localized swelling and distortion of the tissue planes may be the only early findings. Bone destruction is usually not appreciated until 35 to 40% of the involved region is destroyed, and thus is generally not evident for 10 to 14 days (5,7,22). In addition, the degree of involvement is often underestimated on routine radiographs. In this situation, conventional tomography or CT may be useful in more clearly defining the extent of involvement. CT has been especially useful in determining the extent of disease prior to planning operative therapy (20).

Radioisotope studies provide a sensitive tool for early detection of osteomyelitis. Technetium-99m, gallium-67, and indium-111 labeled leukocytes provide sensitive and fairly specific methods for diagnosis of infection (4,5,7,12,15). However, the anatomic extent may be inaccurate, especially in the articular regions, and differentiation of cellulitis from bone involvement is not always possible.

Motion artifact is generally not a problem in the lower extremities. Therefore, MR imaging is particularly suited to evaluate osteomyelitis in these areas. Anatomic detail is superior to that provided by isotope studies, and subtle bone and soft tissue changes are more easily appreciated than on radiographs or CT examinations (2–4,8,11,24). In determining the effectiveness of MR imaging in evaluating infection, the following questions must be answered: (a) Can MR imaging detect infection as early as or earlier than isotope studies? (b) Are image characteristics and/or calculated T1 and T2 changes specific? (c) Can healing and treatment be effectively monitored?

As with other musculoskeletal pathology, examination of patients with infection requires both T1- [partial saturation or inversion recovery (IR)] and T2- [spin–echo with long echo time (TE; ≥60) and repetition time (TR; >2,000)] weighted sequences (29). These sequences are needed to provide the necessary contrast between normal and abnormal tissue and to detect and characterize subtle abnormalities. Partial saturation sequences (short TE ≤ 30, short TR ≤ 500) can be performed quickly and provide high spatial resolution (4,11). Infection will be seen as an area of decreased signal intensity compared to the high signal intensity of normal marrow. Changes in cortical bone, periosteum, and muscle are often less obvious (Fig. 1). IR sequences may detect more subtle changes but images are noisier and scans require more time (TR usually ≥2,000) (Fig. 2). The T2-weighted sequences (TE ≥ 60, TR ≥ 2,000) demonstrate infection as areas of high signal intensity, which is ideal for distinguishing abnormal areas in cortical bone and soft tissues but which can also reduce the contrast of infected

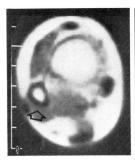
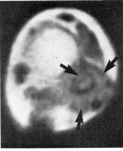

FIG. 1. Osteomyelitis of the distal left fibula. Partial saturation sequence (TE 30, TR 500) demonstrates decreased signal intensity in the medullary bone with similar changes in the periosteum and soft tissues (*black arrows*). Note the normal right fibula (*open arrow*) and similar density of the muscle and soft tissue infection using this sequence. (From Berquist et al., ref. 4, with permission.)

tissue compared to normal marrow (Fig. 3). Infected medullary bone would have a higher intensity than adjacent normal marrow with very long TR values but use of these sequences significantly increases scan time (Table 1). In certain situations, more than two sequences may be required to improve tissue characterization. For example, chemical shift imaging may provide valuable information about fat, water (cellular elements), or inflammatory changes in bone marrow (27).

The anatomic extent of osteomyelitis can be clearly demonstrated by MR imaging (17). The extent of disease, including detection of skip areas, is easily established using transaxial images in combination with either the sagittal or coronal images (see Fig. 11A). This information is particularly valuable in planning surgical debridement. Animal studies have revealed that changes in pathologic specimens correlated well with MR images (Fig. 4).

The specificity of MR imaging in diagnosing osteomyelitis needs to be more clearly defined. Increased signal intensity in marrow, cortical bone, periosteum,

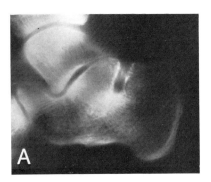
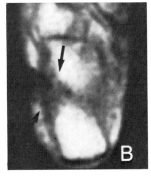

FIG. 2. Osteomyelitis of the calcaneous following osteotomy. **A:** Lateral tomogram of the calcaneous shows the old osteotomy defect but no definite infection. **B:** Axial IR image (TI 500, TE 40, TR 2,000) shows decreased signal (*black arrows*) in the bone and soft tissues due to osteomyelitis. (From Brown et al., ref. 7, with permission.)

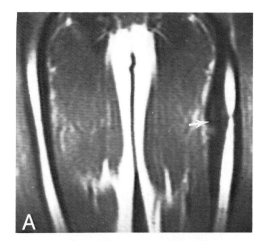

FIG. 3. Chronic osteomyelitis of the left femur. **A:** Coronal partial saturation sequence (TE 30, TR 500) shows thickening of the cortex with gray areas of infection or granulation tissue medially (*arrow*). Axial T2-weighted (TE 60, TR 2,000) spin–echo images (**B, C**) show increased signal in the cortex and medial soft tissues suggesting active infection.

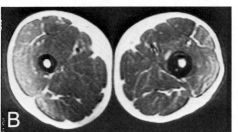

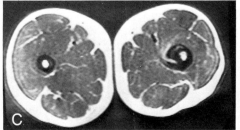

TABLE 1. *MR imaging*

	Imaging features of infection				
	Marrow		Cortical bone		
	Normal	Infection	Normal	Infection	Soft tissues
Partial saturation	White	Dark	Black	Dark (may be slightly gray)	May be difficult to detect
IR	White	Dark	Black	Dark (may be slightly gray)	Signal decreased relative to muscle, nerve, fat
Spin–echo (long TE, TR)	White	White	Black	White	Signal increased relative to muscle; may be similar to fat

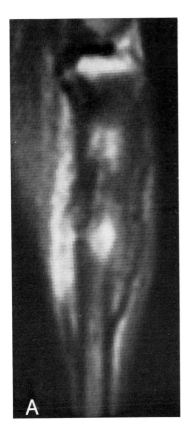

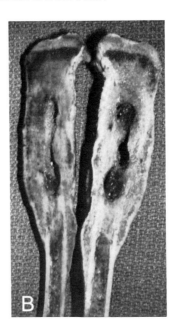

FIG. 4. Osteomyelitis in a dog tibia. Sagittal MR image (**A**) and sagittal section (**B**) of the specimen demonstrating the degree of medullary, cortical and periosteal involvement. (From Petersen et al., ref. 18, with permission.)

and soft tissue is noted on T2-weighted sequences, and decreased signal intensity is evident when a T1-weighted sequence is used. Similar findings, however, have also been noted with neoplasms. The only significant image feature noted to date (T2-weighted sequences) has been increased signal in medullary bone with a well-defined dark margin (4) (Fig. 5). This observation has been noted with both infection and benign tumors (29). Infection must be present for several weeks to allow the reactive region in the medullary bone, which is responsible for this finding, to develop. Calculated T1 and T2 values overlap with other types of pathology (see Table 2 in T. H. Berquist, "Bone and Soft Tissue Tumors," *this volume*). In addition, early studies show that these data do not accurately predict when the infection has been completely eradicated (18).

Despite the sensitivity of MR imaging, certain questions regarding osteomyelitis in nonviolated bone remain unanswered. To date, we have noted that MR images demonstrate changes earlier than radiographs, as well as provide better anatomic

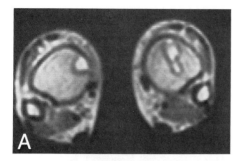

FIG. 5. Osteomyelitis in the tibias **(A)** and right femoral head **(B)**. Note the signal intensity is greater than marrow and that a dark halo is present due to the presence of fiber bone around the infected areas (TE 60, TR 2,000).

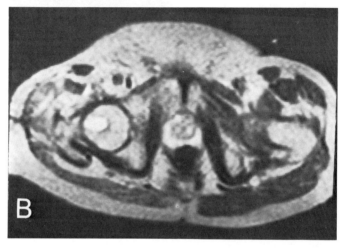

definition (4,11). However, it is not certain if MR imaging can detect abnormalities earlier than radioisotopes (see Fig. 2). By the time that the majority of patients present for evaluation, infections are already well established, and the earliest phase of this process has passed. It is thus difficult to assess the relative usefulness of isotopes and MR imaging. Gallium and indium-111 labeled white blood cells (WBCs) may be more specific; however, anatomic detail is less than that provided by MR imaging.

JOINT SPACE INFECTION

Infectious arthritis is generally monoarticular and, like osteomyelitis, commonly involves the lower extremities (5,7,14). Joint space changes and soft tissue swelling may be noted on radiographs, but early bone changes are not appreciated for 1 to 2 weeks in a pyogenic infection and may take months to develop with tuberculous arthritis (5,14). Isotope scans using technetium-99m are sensitive in detecting early changes, but nonspecific. Gallium and indium-111-WBC scans are more specific in this regard (4,12,15).

The role of MR imaging in joint space infection is unclear. Early bone and soft tissue changes and effusions are easily detected (Fig. 6). However, the findings are not specific and could be noted with many other arthritides. Characterization of the type of fluid present in the joint would be useful. Generally, the T1 and T2 relaxation times of transudates are longer than exudates (9,23). Infected fluid and blood in the joint tend to have an intermediate signal intensity and may be inhomogeneous on T2-weighted images. Normal synovial fluid has a uniformly high signal intensity using this sequence (see Fig. 17 in T. H. Berquist, R. L. Ehman, J. A. Rand, and S. Scott, *this volume*). This information is obviously not sufficient to avoid joint aspiration to identify the offending organism.

SEPTIC SPONDYLITIS

Various terms have been applied to inflammatory changes in the disk space or vertebra. Disk space narrowing with an elevated sedimentation rate has been termed diskitis, infectious diskitis, and intervertebral disk space inflammation (6,7). In adults, the disk is relatively avascular, and infection usually spreads to the disk via the vertebral body rather than the hematogenous route—pyogenic vertebral osteomyelitis (5-7). Septic spondylitis is a general term which includes the spectrum of childhood diskitis and adult vertebral osteomyelitis (7).

Diagnosis of septic spondylitis can be difficult with routine imaging techniques. The first radiographic changes, disk space narrowing with adjacent swelling, may not be evident for several weeks (5). Thus, serial spine films are especially helpful in differentiating septic spondylitis from other causes of disk space narrowing (degenerative, traumatic, etc.). Lucent zones in the adjacent vertebra follow disk narrowing by several weeks, and if left unchecked, progressive collapse and kyphotic deformity can occur (5,7).

Technetium scans may be difficult to interpret, especially in adults with degenerative disease, previous laminectomy, or fusion. Increased accuracy is achieved using Gallium and WBC labeled with indium-111.

CT has played a valuable role in evaluating the disk, vertebra, and surrounding soft tissues. CT guided aspiration is also useful in defining the infecting organism so that the appropriate antibiotics can be used (20). MR imaging, however, can demonstrate changes earlier and more clearly than either CT or routine radiographs (16). This is largely due to the improved soft tissue contrast and the ability

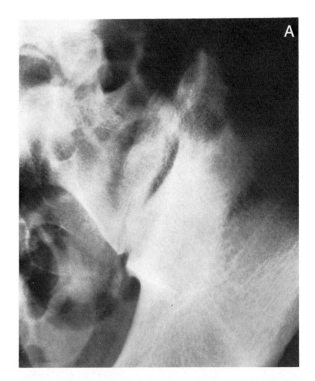

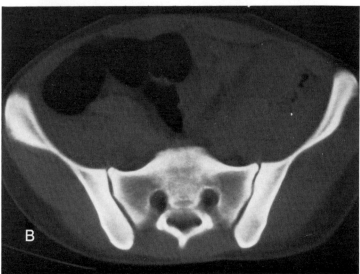

FIG. 6. Infection of the left sacroiliac joint. **A:** Radiograph is normal. **B:** CT scan shows a normal left sacroiliac joint with slight soft tissue asymmetry. **C:** MR image (TR 60, TR 2,000) shows increased intensity in the soft tissues anterior and posterior (*arrows*) to the joint. These findings are not specific for infection but the superior soft tissue contrast clearly demonstrates these inflammatory changes.

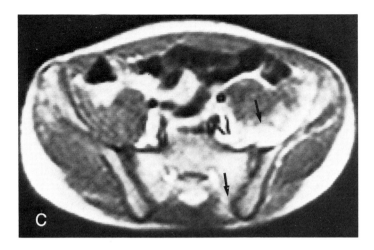

FIG. 6. (*continued.*)

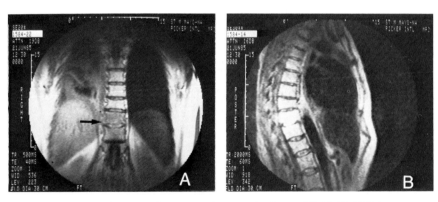

FIG. 7. Disk space infection. **A:** Coronal partial saturation image (TE 40, TR 500) demonstrates decreased signal intensity (*arrow*) in T11–T12 vertebrae with slight paraspinal swelling and right pleural effusion. **B:** Sagittal T2-weighted (TE 60, TR 2,000) image shows marked increase in the signal intensity of the involved disk and adjacent vertebra. Note the compression of T10, T11, and L1.

to perform direct coronal and sagittal imaging (Fig. 7). In a recent review of 37 patients with suspected vertebral osteomyelitis, MR imaging was found to be both accurate and sensitive. Partial saturation sequences (TE 30, TR 500) demonstrated decreased signal in the vertebral bodies and involved disk. T2-weighted spin–echo sequences (TE 120, TR 3,000) revealed higher signal intensity than normal disks or marrow in the involved areas. In addition, sagittal MR images provide a noninvasive means for evaluating kyphotic angulation and the extent of spinal canal involvement (16).

INFECTION IN VIOLATED TISSUE

Detection of infection in patients with violated bone and soft tissue presents a difficult diagnostic problem. This includes patients with previous fracture or surgical intervention, either for fracture reduction or joint replacement. Radiographs and tomograms may be difficult to interpret in the early phases of infection due to the changes of fracture healing. Subtle changes adjacent to metal fixation devices and joint replacements are also not seen for weeks. The usually reliable technetium-99m scan can remain positive for more than 10 months following fracture or surgery, but indium-111-labeled leukocytes and gallium scans have been more successful in these patients (15). The anatomic detail and combination of joint aspiration and anesthetic injection have made subtraction arthrography a very useful exam for patients with joint replacement and suspected infection (7).

In a review of the MR imaging studies in over 50 patients with infection in violated bone and soft tissues, we observed abnormalities in all examinations. However, in many cases it was difficult to differentiate areas of osteomyelitis from zones of fracture healing. Fracture healing results in cortical thickening with granulation tissue and fibrocartilage in the region of the fracture. The T2-weighted images are most useful because they provide the best contrast between cortical bone and granulation tissue or fibrocartilage. Subtle changes in medullary bone can be seen with IR or sequences with short TE and TR. Areas of potential infection tend to have longer T2 relaxation times due to increased free water content compared to the areas of healing (Fig. 8). Hemorrhage also has a long T2, but at low and medium field strengths the T2 shortens over a 10 to 17 day period which may assist in differentiating hemorrhage or hematoma from untreated areas of infection (21).

Routine radiographs or tomography are clearly very useful for identifying sequestra, which appear as areas of decreased signal on MR images. The artifact created by metal implants (on MR images), though often minimal, may prohibit evaluation of subtle bone changes immediately adjacent to the metal (Figs. 9 and 10). However, we have found that periosteal changes and soft tissue abnor-

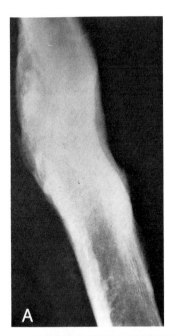

FIG. 8. Femoral osteomyelitis following fracture. **A:** Radiograph demonstrating old fracture deformity with sclerosis and cortical thickening. **B:** Axial MR image (TE 60, TR 2,000) shows cortical irregularity on the right with granulation tissue (*arrow*) and increased signal intensity (*open arrow*) which may be infection or normal marrow. There is increased signal in the soft tissues with a cutaneous defect suggesting infection.

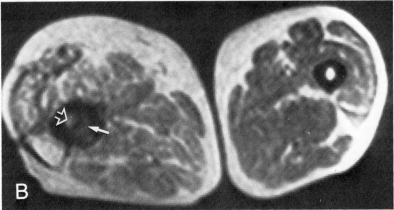

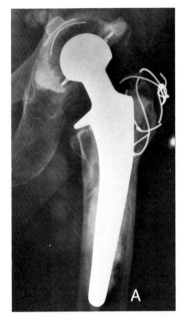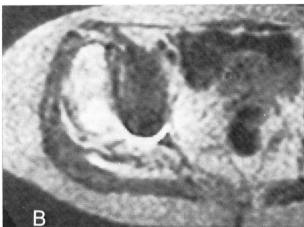

FIG. 9. Soft tissue infection following total hip arthroplasty. **A:** Radiograph demonstrating THA with no evidence of infection or loosening. **B:** Axial (TE 120, TR 2,000) image demonstrating in a localized collection of inhomogeneous fluid adjacent to the hip. Note the artifact does not allow assessment of the bone immediately adjacent to the metal.

malities can be easily detected even in the region of the hip, where the amount and configuration of the metal tends to cause more artifact.

SURGICAL RECONSTRUCTION

A high percentage of adult patients with chronic osteomyelitis require surgical therapy for excision of necrotic or infected tissue. The use of free vascularized

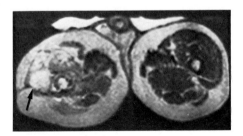

FIG. 10. Old fracture of the upper right femur. There is a soft tissue abscess (*arrow*) with a sinus tract in the subcutaneous tissues.

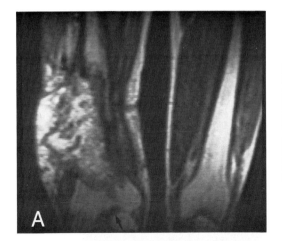

FIG. 11. Chronic osteomyelitis of the distal femur with vascularized omental graft. The coronal (**A**) and axial (**B**) (TE 30, TR 500) MR images show that the graft fills the dead space. The omental fat has high signal intensity and appears viable. There is an area of decreased intensity in the distal femur (*arrow*) representing a separate area of potential infection.

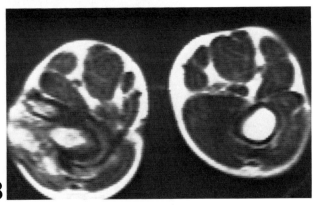

muscle and omental and bone grafts is increasing in the treatment of patients with chronic osteomyelitis (1,10,13,25,26,28). Reconstructive procedures may be needed depending on the vascularity of adjacent tissue and the size and type of defect (26). There are several basic goals regardless of the tissue or technique used. These include (a) wound coverage, (b) obliteration of dead space (which may permit survival of existing organisms or provide a medium for recurrent infection), and (c) provide optimal vascular supply to the described area (25,26,28).

Preoperative assessment should include review of the necessary information and planning of the surgical approach; postoperative assessment should determine whether or not the surgical goals have been achieved. Preoperatively, MR imaging is an ideal way to assess the extent of bone and soft tissue involvement, as well

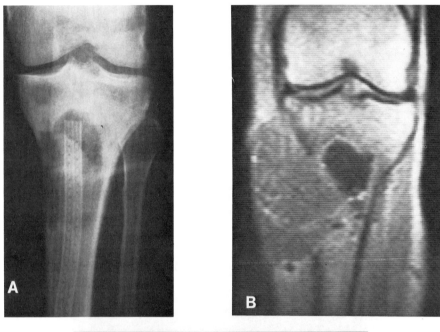

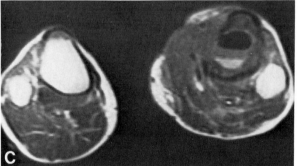

FIG. 12.   Osteomyelitis of the proximal tibia treated with muscle flap. **A:** anteroposterior radiograph showing the bone defect in the upper tibia. Coronal (**B**), axial (**C**), and sagittal (**D**) MR images using partial saturation techniques show a large residual dead space with air, blood, and fluid in the dead space. This is an ideal medium for recurrent infection. The patient was returned to surgery and the dead space (**E**) filled by repositioning the flap.

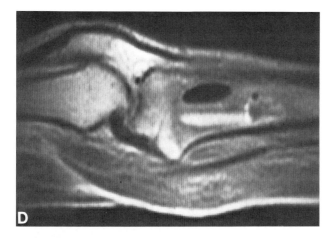

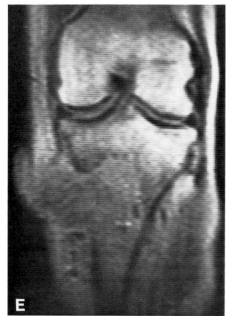

FIG. 12. (*continued.*)

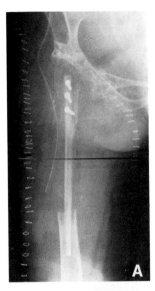

FIG. 13. Fibular graft upper right femur. **A:** Radiograph demonstrates the position of the fibular graft in the upper femur with screws proximally and numerous surgical staples. **B:** Axial MR image demonstrates the graft (*arrow*) with normal surrounding musculature.

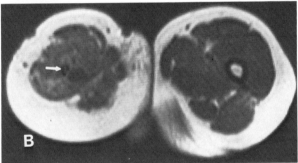

as to detect skip areas. Preoperative images also serve as a valuable base line to later determine whether the surgical goals are achieved (Fig. 11).

MR imaging is well suited to evaluate defect coverage or dead space, residual infection, and hematomas or fluid collections which may serve as media for recurrent infection (Fig. 12). MR imaging is particularly useful in the evaluation of omental (Fig. 11) and muscle flaps (Fig. 12). Vascularized fibular grafts can be evaluated, but the small amount of marrow presents certain problems (Fig. 13), as there is little fibular marrow to image in the axial plane. This can be improved by using coronal and sagittal views, which increase the marrow volume imaged and allow the position as well as the proximal and distal attachments of the grafts to be more easily evaluated (Fig. 14).

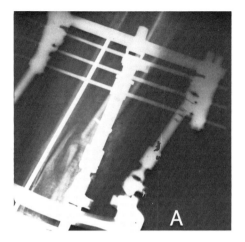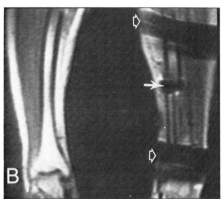

FIG. 14. Fibular graft in the distal tibia. **A:** Radiograph of the tibia with Ace–Fisher fixateur. **B:** Coronal (TE 40, TR 500) MR image shows the fibular graft in good position. Note the bone formation (*arrow*) at the proximal end. Areas of no signal (*open arrows*) due to the fixation device.

Further studies and follow-up of these patients will be needed to determine the effectiveness of MR imaging in evaluating viability and flow factors in the grafts. Spectroscopy may also play a role in graft evaluation, especially early ischemic changes.

REFERENCES

1. Arnold, P. G., and Irons, G. B. (1984): Lower extremity muscle flaps. *Orthop. Clin. North Am.,* 15:441–449.
2. Baker, H. L., Jr., Berquist, T. H., Kispert, D. B., Reese, D. F., Houser, O. W., Earnest, F., IV, Forbes, G. S., and May, G. R. (1985): Magnetic resonance imaging in a routine clinical setting. *Mayo Clin. Proc.,* 60:75–90.
3. Berquist, T. H. (1984): Magnetic resonance imaging: Preliminary experience in orthopedic radiology. *Magnetic Resonance Imaging,* 2:41–52.
4. Berquist, T. H., Brown, M. L., Fitzgerald, R. H., Jr., and May, G. R. (1985): Magnetic resonance imaging: Application in musculoskeletal infection. *Magnetic Resonance Imaging,* 3:219–230.
5. Bonakdapour, A., and Gaines, V. D. (1983): The radiology of osteomyelitis. *Orthop. Clin. North Am.,* 14:21–37.
6. Boston, H. C., Bianco, A. J., Jr., and Rhodes, K. H. (1975): Disk space infections in children. *Orthop. Clin. North Am.,* 6:953–964.
7. Brown, M. L., Kamida, C. B., Berquist, T. H., and Fitzgerald, R. H., Jr. (1986): An imaging approach to musculoskeletal infections. In: *Imaging of Orthopedic Trauma and Surgery,* edited by T. H. Berquist, pp. 731–753. W.B. Saunders, Philadelphia.
8. Cohen, M. D., Klatte, E. C., Baehner, R., Smith, J. A., Martin-Simmerman, P., Carr, B. E., Provisor, A. J., Weetman, R. M., Coates, T., Siddiqui, A., Weisman, S. J., Berkow, R., McKenna, S., and McGuire, W. A. (1984): Magnetic resonance imaging of bone marrow disease in children. *Radiology,* 151:715–718.

9. Cophen, J. M., Weinreb, J. C., and Maravilla, K. R. (1985): Fluid collections in the intraperitoneal and extraperitoneal spaces: Comparison of MR and CT. *Radiology.* 155:705–708.

10. Fitzgerald, R. H., Ruttle, P. E., Arnold, P. G., Kelly, P. J., and Irons, G. B. (1985): Local muscle flaps in the treatment of chronic osteomyelitis. *J. Bone Joint Surg. [Am.]*, 67:175–185.

11. Fletcher, B. D., Scoles, P. V., and Nelson, A. D. (1984): Osteomyelitis in children: Detection by magnetic resonance. *Radiology,* 150:57–60.

12. Howie, D. W., Savage, J. P., and Wilson, T. G. (1983): The technetium phosphate bone scan in the diagnosis of osteomyelitis in children. *J. Bone Joint Surg. [Am.]*, 65:431–437.

13. Irons, G. B., Fisher, J., and Schmitt, E. H. (1984): Vascularized muscular and musculocutaneous flaps for management of osteomyelitis. *Orthop. Clin. North Am.,* 15:473–480.

14. Kelly, P. J., Martin, W. J., and Coventry, M. B. (1970): Bacterial arthritis in the adult. *J. Bone Joint Surg. [Am.]*, 52:1595–1602.

15. Merkel, K. D., Brown, M. L., Dewanjee, M. K., and Fitzgerald, R. H., Jr. (1985): Comparison of indium-labeled leukocyte imaging with sequential technetium-gallium scanning in diagnosis low-grade musculoskeletal sepsis: A prospective study. *J. Bone Joint Surg. [Am.]*, 67:465–476.

16. Modic, M. T., Feiglin, D. H., Piraino, D. W., Boumphrey, F., Weinstein, M. A., Duchesneau, P. M., and Rehm, S. (1985): Veterbral osteomyelitis: Assessment using MR. *Radiology,* 157: 157–166.

17. Moon, K. L., Jr., Genant, H. G., Helms, C. A., Chafetz, N. I., Crooks, L. E., and Kaufman, L. (1983): Musculoskeletal applications of nuclear magnetic resonance. *Radiology,* 147:161–171.

18. Petersen, S. A., Berquist, T. H., and Fitzgerald, R. H., Jr. (1986): Magnetic resonance imaging in musculoskeletal sepsis (*in press*).

19. Scott, J. A., Rosenthal, D. I., and Brady, T. J. (1984): The evaluation of musculoskeletal disease with magnetic resonance imaging. *Radiol. Clin. North Am.,* 22:917–924.

20. Seltzer, S. E. (1984): Value of computed tomography in planning medical and surgical treatment of chronic osteomyelitis. *J. Comput. Assist. Tomogr.,* 8:482–487.

21. Swensen, S. J., Keller, P. L., Berquist, T. H., McLeod, R. A., and Stephens, D. H. (1985): Magnetic resonance of hemorrhage. *A. J. R.,* 145:921–927.

22. Waldvogel, F. A., Medoff, G., and Sehwartz, M. N. (1970): Osteomyelitis: A review of clinical features, therapeutic considerations, and unusual aspects. *N. Engl. J. Med.,* 282:198–206.

23. Wall, S. D., Fisher, M. R., Amparo, E. G., Hricak, H., and Higgins, C. B. (1985): Magnetic resonance imaging in the evaluation of abscesses. *A. J. R.,* 144:1217–1221.

24. Weekes, R. G., Berquist, T. H., McLeod, R. A., and Zimmer, W. D. (1985): Magnetic resonance imaging of soft tissue tumors: Comparison with computed tomography. *Magnetic Resonance Imaging,* 3(4):345–352.

25. Weiland, A. J. (1985): Symposium: The use of muscle flaps in the treatment of osteomyelitis in the lower extremity. *Contemporary Orthopaedics,* 10:127–159.

26. Weiland, A. J., Moore, J. R., and David, R. K. (1984): The efficacy of free tissue transfer in treatment of osteomyelitis. *J. Bone Joint Surg. [Am.]*, 66:181–193.

27. Wismer, G. L., Rosen, B. R., Buxton, R., Start, D. D., and Brady, T. J. (1985): Chemical shift imaging of bone marrow: Preliminary experience. *A. J. R.,* 145:1031–1037.

28. Wood, M. B., and Cooney, W. P., III (1984): Vascularized bone segment transfers for management of chronic osteomyelitis. *Orthop. Clin. North Am.,* 15:401–472.

29. Zimmer, W. D., Berquist, T. H., McLeod, R. A., Sim, F. H., Pritchard, D. J., Shives, T. C., Wold, L. E., and May, G. R. (1985): Bone tumors: MRI vs. CT. *Radiology,* 155:709–718.

Musculoskeletal Trauma

Thomas H. Berquist, Richard L. Ehman,
*James A. Rand, and †Steven Scott

*Mayo Medical School, and Departments of Diagnostic Radiology, *Orthopedic Surgery,
and †Physical Medicine and Rehabilitation, Mayo Clinic, Rochester, Minnesota 55905*

The number of musculoskeletal injuries related to sports and other recreational activities has steadily increased. This is due, in part, to increased participation in organized sports and renewed interest in physical fitness (9,10,22,24,32,43,44,47). Early detection of the type and extent of musculoskeletal injury is essential for planning proper management (25,32).

TYPES OF INJURY

Skeletal injuries (complete and incomplete fractures, stress fractures, insufficiency fractures, etc.) are common. Diagnosis of these injuries is generally possible with routine radiography, conventional or computed tomography (CT), and isotope scans (16,17,19,20,38,46,56,57). Evaluation of soft tissue injury is more difficult, particularly deep soft tissue injury (32,45). Soft tissue techniques, including xerography, low kilovolt peak (kVp) radiographs, and invasive modalities such as arthrography, bursography, and tenography are successful in certain situations (7,15). Magnetic resonance (MR) imaging has demonstrated significant potential for evaluation of soft tissue trauma (6,29). MR imaging provides excellent soft tissue contrast, and images can be obtained in the transaxial, coronal, and sagittal planes (11). These two factors allow detection of subtle soft tissue changes and the extent of involvement following injury (8,25,48).

Understanding the changes which occur with bone and soft tissue injury is essential to determine the best imaging technique. Soft tissue contusions occur following a direct blow, resulting in capillary rupture with local infiltrative hemorrhage followed by edema and inflammation. Hematomas, or more confined collections of blood, may also develop (32).

Muscles, ligaments, and tendons may rupture due to direct or indirect trauma (forceful muscle contraction). Disruption may occur acutely or result from recurrent injury or incomplete healing (25). The terms "sprain" and "strain" are used to describe these soft tissue injuries. The subcommittee on athletic nomenclature of the American Medical Association suggests the term strain be applied to muscle–tendon units and sprain to ligaments (32). Determination of the degree of injury to either of these units is essential in treatment planning. Ligament sprains (Fig. 1) have been classified as follows: first degree: disruption of only a few fibers; second degree: disruption of a significant number of ligament fibers, but sparing at least 50% of the ligament; and third degree: complete disruption of the ligament. A fourth category, fracture/sprain, has been used to describe avulsion fractures. Strains, injuries to muscle–tendon units, are similarly described as first to third degree depending upon the degree of disruption of the muscle or tendon (3,32). During the healing process, certain physiological changes occur which can be easily monitored with MR imaging. During the acute phase (first week) there is edema and hemorrhage or hematoma formation. In the second week fibroblast proliferation occurs. Organization and granulation tissue formation takes place in the third to sixth weeks after injury. Further organization and subsequent healing may take more than 12 weeks (2,32) (Figs. 9 and 10).

Stress syndrome, tenosynovitis, and bursitis are commonly caused by chronic overuse. In the two latter cases, inflammation leads to increased synovial fluid, influx of inflammatory cells, and local hyperemia (24,32).

MR imaging is ideal for evaluating these post-traumatic soft tissue changes. Swensen et al. (51) studied hemorrhage and hematoma formation (0.15-T magnet) using phantoms with blood samples, animal models, and patients with known post-traumatic hematomas. In the acute setting the majority of hematomas ap-

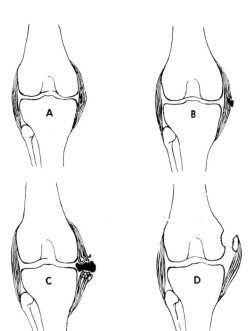

FIG. 1. Classification of ligament injuries using the medial collateral ligament as a model. **A:** First degree sprain. **B:** Second degree sprain. **C:** Third degree sprain, and **D:** sprain-fracture. (From O'Donoghue, ref. 32, with permission.)

peared dark [long longitudinal relaxation time (T1) > 543 msec, at 0.15 T (tesla)] on T1-weighted sequences [inversion recovery (IR), inversion time (TI) 400, relaxation time (TR) 2,100] and were high signal intensity or white on transverse relaxation time (T2) [spin–echo echo time (TE) 80, TR 2,100] weighted sequences. With time, the hematomas organized. Over a 16-day period there was a gradual decrease in both T1 and T2 with resulting increased intensity on T1-weighted images and decreased intensity on T2 images (Fig. 2). The density of hematomas was increased above that of normal muscle on partial saturation image (SE, TE 40, TR 500). Changes noted with infiltrative hemorrhage were similar, but the decrease in T1 and T2 occurred more slowly. It should be noted that the appearance of hemorrhage at higher field strengths (1.5 T) may differ significantly (see R. L. Ehman, *this volume*).

Variations in anatomy and clinical indication may result in significantly different approaches using MR imaging techniques. Therefore, discussion of MR

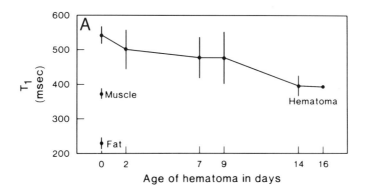

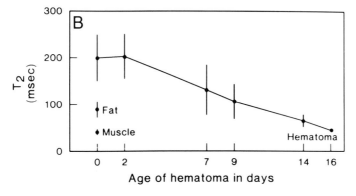

FIG. 2. Graphs demonstrating gradual decrease in T1 (**A**) and T2 (**B**) of hematomas over a 16-day period. The normal T1 and T2 of fat and muscle are provided for comparison. (From Swensen et al., ref. 51, with permission.)

imaging applications in evaluation of trauma is facilitated by using an anatomic approach.

Spine

MR imaging of the spine will be thoroughly discussed elsewhere (M. L. Richardson, *this volume*). However, we will briefly discuss the potential applications of MR imaging in evaluation of spinal trauma.

Fractures and fracture dislocations of the spine can usually be detected with routine radiography. In certain situations (facet and odontoid fractures) tomography may be required. CT is particularly useful in evaluating the position of bone fragments in the spinal canal. When combined with metrizamide myelography, the cord and epidural space can also be effectively evaluated with CT. These techniques are well suited to the severely injured patient because the examinations can be quickly accomplished and there is better access to the patient if life support equipment is needed (7,8).

Currently, MR imaging is not often used to evaluate patients with severe or unstable spinal injuries. However, MR imaging may provide certain advantages in clinically stable patients or patients with suspected spinal or perispinal soft tissue injuries. MR imaging allows direct visualization of the spinal canal and cord (Figs. 3 and 4), and displacement, swelling, and intra- or extramedullary hematomas of the cord can be easily detected (35). These findings can be evaluated quickly using multisection direct sagittal views. Fractures may be identified as areas of increased signal in cortical bone (T2-weighted images), decreased signal in medullary bone (T1-weighted images) (Fig. 3), or by compression or anatomic configuration change in the vertebral body. Disc abnormalities are also easily identified (27,28,30) (Fig. 4).

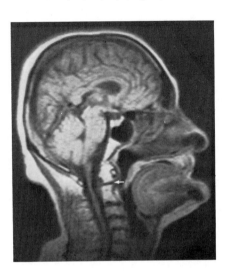

FIG. 3. Sagittal image of the upper cervical spine. The cord and spinal canal are clearly demonstrated. A type II odontoid fracture (*arrow*) is seen as an area of decreased signal intensity (TE 30, TR 500).

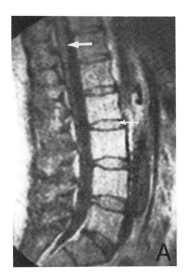
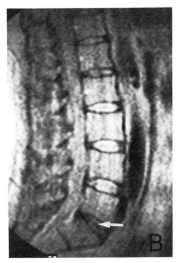

FIG. 4. Sagittal images of the lumbar spine using short and long TR. **A:** Spin–echo (TE 40, TR 500) shows the nucleus pulposus has higher signal intensity than the annulus and cortical bone. The cerebrospinal fluid is black and cord (*large arrow*) intermediate intensity. **B:** Increasing the TR to 4,000 causes the intensity of the cerebrospinal fluid to increase, obscuring the cord. The signal intensity of the normal disks increase, allowing degenerative changes (*arrow*) and other abnormalities of the disk to be more easily detected.

Detection of soft tissue injury in paraspinal muscles or posterior supporting ligaments is also a potential application of MR imaging (Fig. 5). These soft tissue injuries are difficult to evaluate with conventional techniques; fluoroscopically monitored flexion and extension views are helpful in evaluating soft tissue injury and stability but are often inaccurate in the acute setting (7). The soft tissue contrast of MR imaging is superior to CT and other imaging techniques in detection of hematoma and other post-traumatic changes. This fact has been demonstrated with MR imaging in the extremities (6,8,29,52).

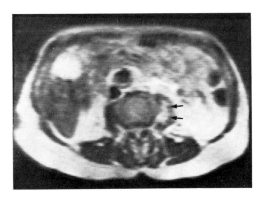

FIG. 5. Axial image of the lumbar spine. There is hemorrhage (*arrow*) in the left psoas muscle due to trauma. Acute hemorrhage has increased signal intensity on T2-weighted images (TE > 60, TR > 2,000; 0.15 T).

The imaging sequences and planes should be tailored to the type of spinal or paraspinal pathology suspected. As discussed previously (T. H. Berquist, "Technical Considerations in Magnetic Resonance Imaging," *this volume*), both T1- and T2-weighted sequences are usually required to provide the necessary information. One sequence can be performed in the transaxial plane and the other in either the coronal or the sagittal plane. For examination of the cord, discs, and vertebral bodies (shape, alignment, etc.) the sagittal plane is most often used. Pulse sequences with short TE and TR can be performed quickly (4.5 min using four averages and a 500 msec repetition time) and provide excellent detail. Subtle soft tissue hemorrhage or disc changes may be overlooked with this sequence. Therefore, a more T2-weighted sequence should also be performed (TE > 60, TR > 2,000). Sequences with long TE and TR also increase the signal intensity of the cerebral spinal fluid (Fig. 4). This provides an appearance similar to a myelogram, but the cord is often obscured in the process. Table 1 summarizes the advantages and disadvantages of MR imaging in evaluation of the spine and paraspinal tissues. The major disadvantages (scan time, spatial resolution, and partial volume effects due to slice thickness) have been improved with new software, surface coil technology, and increased field strength. Larger field strengths, 1 to 2 T, are now available. These units increase the signal-to-noise ratio and allow fewer averages (decrease exam time) and thinner slices (27).

Pelvis, Hips, and Thighs

Musculoskeletal injuries are particularly common in the pelvis, hips, and lower extremities and are often sports related. Twenty-five to thirty million Americans jog or run regularly; McKeag reported 1,800 injuries in 16,000 runners over only a 2-year period (24).

TABLE 1. *MR imaging of spinal and paraspinal trauma*

Advantages	Disadvantages
Direct cord visualization	Poor spatial resolution[a]
Noninvasive	Long scan time[a]
Direct coronal and sagittal images	Slice thickness[a]
Soft tissue contrast	Patient limitations
No cortical bone artifact	aneurysm clips
	pacemakers
	scoliosis
	Miss cortical bone fragments

[a] These problems should be solved with increased field strength and surface coil technology.
Data from refs. 26, 28, 30, and 35.

Skeletal trauma is still most accurately evaluated with conventional techniques. Evaluation of complex pelvic fractures is better accomplished with CT; other pelvic fractures such as stress fractures or insufficiency fractures are detected most easily with isotope scans (9,16,17,19,37,46,57). The excellent soft tissue contrast provided by MR imaging allows differentiation of muscle, fat, nerves, and blood vessels without the use of contrast material (Fig. 6). Therefore, MR imaging is most effective in evaluation of soft tissue injury or complications of trauma such as avascular necrosis of the femoral head (Fig. 7).

Injuries to thigh muscles or their pelvic insertions are common in trained and untrained athletes. Renstrom (43) reported that 30% of all soccer injuries were either hematomas or muscle strains in the thigh. The hamstring muscles are injured most frequently (3,29,31,32) (Fig. 8), but tears in the quadriceps (Fig. 9) and adductor muscles also occur. Patients usually present with pain and localized swelling, the extent of injury ranging from simple contusion to complete disruption of the muscle–tendon unit. Direct or indirect nerve involvement may result in femoral or sciatic nerve palsies. Fortunately, most injuries are either first or second degree strains, but even then, healing may take as long as 20 weeks (3,42).

Compartment syndromes are more common in the lower leg but have been reported in the posterior thigh (39). Patients present with pain, decreased function, and circulatory compromise due to increased pressure. Ischemic changes may progress if not diagnosed early, and in patients with recurrent compartment syndrome, necrosis and/or fibrous replacement may occur (32,39).

Determination of the degree of injury is important in treatment planning. In addition to evaluation of the acute injury, MR imaging provides a useful tool for following patients undergoing conservative management (Fig. 10). MR imaging is also useful to exclude other pathology which may mimic muscle injury, including infected hematomas, neoplasms, atrophy, etc. (Figs. 11 and 12).

The pelvis and upper thighs are usually examined in the body or close-fitting saddle coils (see Fig. 8 in T. H. Berquist, "Technical Considerations in Magnetic Resonance Imaging," *this volume*). The patient is supine unless the gluteal muscles or muscles of the posterior thigh are being examined, when the prone position prevents distortion of the posterior soft tissues. Examination of the distal thighs can usually be performed using the smaller head coil. In general, the smallest coil possible should be used to obtain better image quality. We routinely use the transaxial and coronal planes to examine the pelvis, hips, and thighs; coronal images allow comparison of the involved and uninvolved extremity. As previously mentioned, both T1- and T2-weighted sequences should be used.

Knee

Knee injuries are common in all age groups. Diagnosis of fractures and dislocation is usually not difficult with current techniques. In selected cases surface

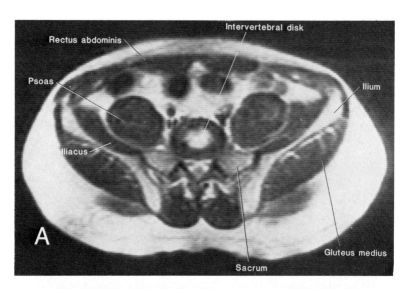

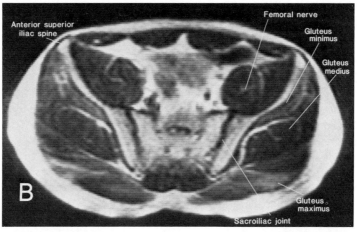

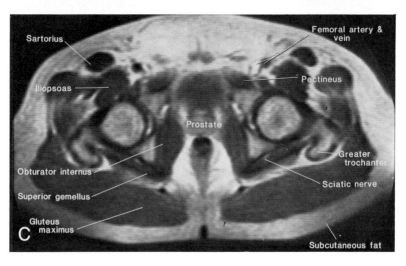

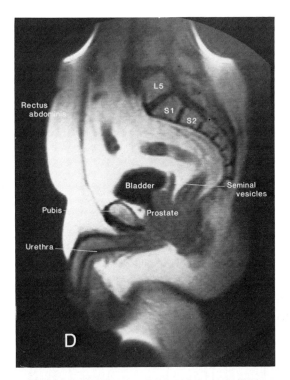

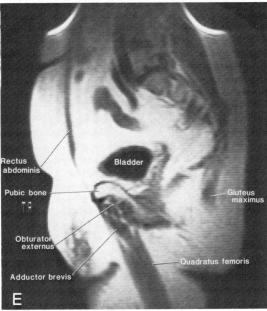

FIG. 6. Normal pelvis anatomy (TR 40, TE 500). **A:** Transaxial image through the upper pelvis at the lumbosacral level. **B:** Transaxial image through the mid sacrum. **C:** Transaxial image through the hips at the level of the greater trochanter. Midline (**D**) and off-midline (**E**) sagittal images of the pelvis.

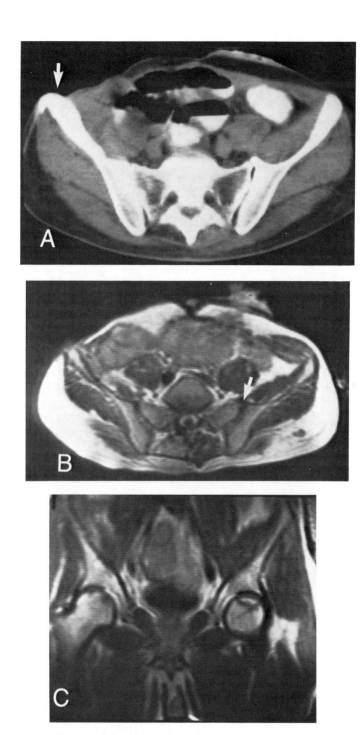

FIG. 7. Patient with a previous pelvic fracture and suspected infection of the ilium due to an open wound. **A:** CT scan through the anterior superior iliac spine demonstrates the defect over the ilium (*arrow*). **B:** Axial MR image shows no evidence of osteomyelitis, but there is widening of the sacroiliac joint (*arrow*) due to the previous fracture. Coronal image (**C**) demonstrates bilateral avascular necrosis of the femoral heads.

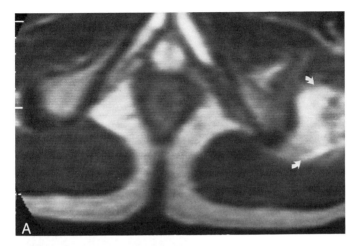

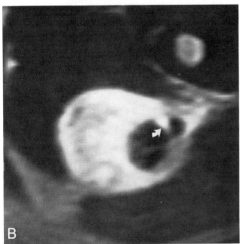

FIG. 8. Hamstring tear near the ischial origin. Routine transaxial (**A**) and localized view (**B**) (TE 60, TR 2,000) demonstrate increased signal intensity near the ischial tuberosity due to hemorrhage. The tendons (dark in **B**) also demonstrate partial tears with hemorrhage (*arrow*). Second degree strain.

FIG. 9. Transaxial image of the thigh in a patient with a healing tear in the rectus femoris. There is also slight muscle atrophy in the involved leg.

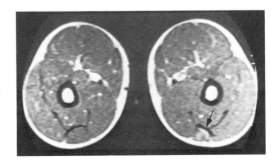

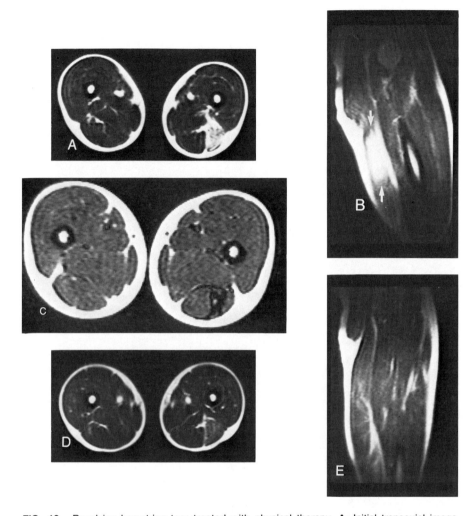

FIG. 10. Resolving hamstring tear treated with physical therapy. **A:** Initial transaxial image (TE 60, TR 2,000) demonstrates a high signal intensity area due to a tear in the biceps femoris muscle. **B:** Sagittal views demonstrate the degree of muscle involvement (*arrows*). **C:** A T1-weighted image (IR, TI 400, TR 1,500) shows the acute hemorrhage as a black density allowing this to be differentiated from fat. Follow-up images (**D** and **E**) 2 weeks after treatment demonstrate that the signal intensity of the hemorrhage is decreasing and the area of involvement is reduced.

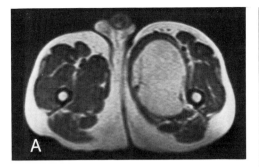
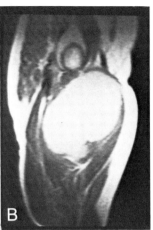

FIG. 11. Patient with clinically suspected adductor tear. Transaxial (**A**) and sagittal (**B**) images demonstrate a large high intensity mass (TE 60, TR 2,000) consistent with a cystic structure. Pathology: benign epithelial lined cyst.

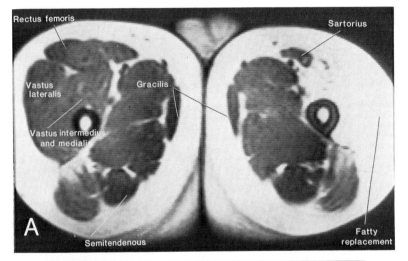

FIG. 12. Patient with long-standing neuropathy and thigh pain. Transaxial (**A**) and coronal (**B**) images demonstrate complete fatty replacement of the vastus lateralis and intermedius.

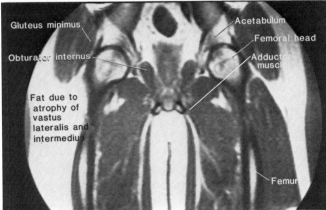

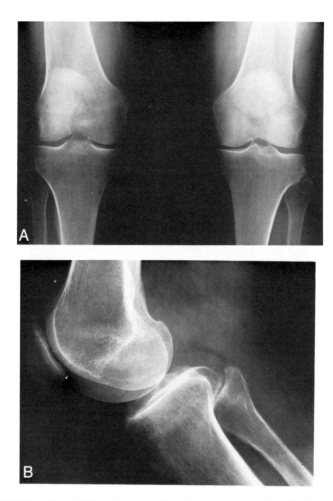

FIG. 13. AP (**A**) and lateral (**B**) radiographs of the knee were normal in this elderly patient with knee pain. MR surface coil images (TE 30, TR 600; 1.5 T) in the axial (**C**) and sagittal (**D**) planes show small insufficiency fractures (*arrows*).

coil images have detected or clarified suspicious skeletal findings (Fig. 13). Soft tissue injuries can be difficult to evaluate, especially with the pain and swelling which accompany acute injury. The accuracy of clinical evaluation approaches 70% (2,40,58). Routine radiographs, stress views, and arthrography can also be inaccurate in this clinical setting (7,8,36,53). Arthrography is 60 to 91% effective and arthroscopy 73 to 97% effective in accurately evaluating knee injuries (2,8,40). Both techniques are limited to intracapsular structures. With arthrography, the cruciate ligaments are more difficult to evaluate than the menisci, and even with arthroscopy, a torn or partially torn cruciate may be hidden by the intact synovial

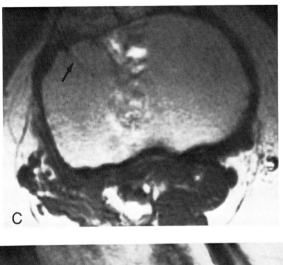

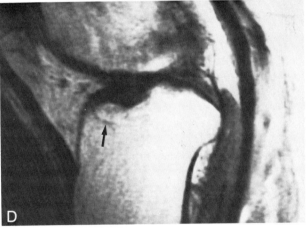

FIG. 13. (*continued.*)

sheath (34,43,54). The extracapsular ligaments and muscle–tendon support units can only be evaluated on the basis of indirect findings (Table 2).

Knee injuries are among the most potentially disabling athletic injuries, making it essential that the diagnosis and treatment be established early. Delay may lead to early osteoarthritis and instability (2). MR imaging has demonstrated significant potential in evaluating the intra- and extracapsular structures of the knee (Table 2).

MR examinations of the knee vary depending on the suspected site of involvement (23,41,42) (Table 3). For purposes of discussion the examinations can be categorized as extra- and intracapsular.

TABLE 2. *Evaluation of the knee structures and techniques*

Structures	Arthrography	Arthroscopy	MR imaging
Menisci	+	+	+
Cruciate ligament			
Anterior	±	+	±
Posterior	±	+	+
Capsule	+	+	±
Synovium	+ (D/C)	+	±
Articular surfaces	+ (D/C)	+	+
Collateral ligaments			
Medial	±	±	+
Lateral	−	−	+
Muscles	−	−	+
Patellar ligaments	−	−	+
Quadriceps	−	−	+

+, Acceptable technique; ±, potential application or occasionally useful; −, not useful; D/C, double contrast technique.

Extracapsular Structures

Examination of the muscles, quadriceps tendon, patellar ligament, and collateral ligaments may be accomplished in the prone or supine position. The patient should be prone if the posterior musculature is the major area of interest. Coil selection depends on whether comparison with the uninvolved extremity is necessary. If not, the smaller knee coil or surface coils can be used (Fig. 14) which improves the signal-to-noise ratio resulting in superior image quality. The amount of sagittal offset should also be considered: if the smaller head coil is used (both knees in the coil) the amount of sagittal offset available may not allow sagittal views through the midpoint of both knees. In this situation the knees may have to be repositioned or examined separately with surface coils.

The midline structures—quadriceps tendon and patellar ligament—are most easily demonstrated with sagittal and transaxial views (Fig. 15). The knee should be positioned with the patella anteriorly. Injuries to these ligaments are easily

TABLE 3. *MR imaging examination of the knee*

Structure	Image plane
Patellar ligament	Sagittal and axial
Quadriceps tendon	Sagittal and axial
Cruciate ligaments	Sagittal (oblique)
Menisci	Coronal and sagittal
Collateral ligaments	Coronal and axial

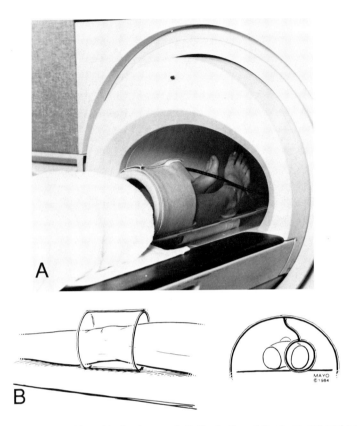

FIG. 14. A: Patient positioned in the knee coil. **B:** Illustration of the knee coil and position of the knee in the magnet (*inset*). With current software, the knee should be shifted to the center of the coil to obtain optimal image quality. This will not be necessary when software for off-axis field of view is available.

demonstrated using a partial saturation sequence in the sagittal plane (four or more sections, TE 30, TR 500) and a T2-weighted sequence in the axial plane (eight to 16 sections, TE 60, TR 2,000). This examination can be completed in less than 25 min (Figs. 16 and 17). The coronal and axial planes are best suited for examination of the collateral ligaments (Table 3; Fig. 15C). The same sequences and scan time generally apply.

Intracapsular Structures

Joint effusions can usually be detected on lateral radiographs or with ultrasound. Effusions can also be detected using MR imaging. The appearance of the fluid depends on the nature of the fluid and the pulse sequence used (Fig. 18). Typically, synovial fluid appears white on spin–echo sequences with long TE

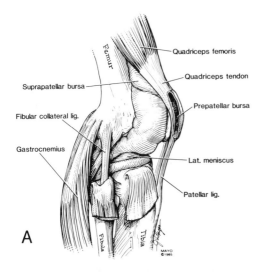

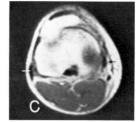

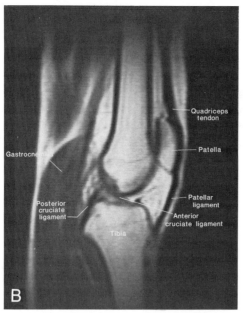

FIG. 15. Normal anatomy of the knee. **A:** Sagittal illustration of the knee. **B:** Midline sagittal MR image (TE 40, TR 500). **C:** Transaxial image through the joint. Note the medial (*black arrow*) and lateral collateral ligaments (*white arrow*). The menisci are not identified.

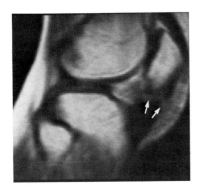

FIG. 16. Sagittal view of the knee (TE 40, TR 500) demonstrating a tear in the patellar ligament (*arrows*). Note the decreased signal of the infrapatellar fat due to edema and hemorrhage (compare Fig. 14).

and TR (TE ≥ 60, TR ≥ 2,000), black on IR, and about the same intensity as muscle with TE 30, TR 500. Bloody effusions tend to have higher intensity with inversion recovery and slightly lower intensity on T2-weighted spin–echo images. To date, we do not have sufficient experience with various causes of effusions (infection, specific arthritides, etc.) to determine if MR imaging can provide specific information about the etiology.

The cruciate ligaments and menisci are more difficult to evaluate than the periarticular structures. Coronal and sagittal images are currently used to evaluate the menisci (Fig. 19), as it is difficult to obtain transaxial images that include the entire meniscus. This is due to the angle of the tibial articular surface (Fig. 15A). Positioning also differs from conventional arthrography. Stressing the knee is not possible due to coil size and inability to maintain a motionless stressed position for the length of time required to obtain the image. Lower field magnets (0.15 T), even with surface coils, do not provide the necessary spatial resolution to detect subtle meniscal lesions (Figs. 19 and 20). The latter problem has been largely solved by using surface coils at higher field strength (1.5 T) and using thinner slices. Currently, arthrography and arthroscopy are more accepted for evaluation of meniscal injuries.

The cruciate ligaments may also be difficult to image. The posterior cruciate ligament is larger than the anterior and extends from the posterior tibial surface in a nearly true sagittal plane to insert in the medial femoral condyle (Fig. 21).

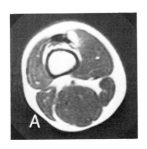
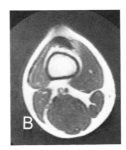

FIG. 17. Patient with knee pain and suspected quadriceps tear. **A:** Axial image (TE 60, TR 2,000) demonstrates increased signal (*arrow*) adjacent to the quadriceps tendon due to a partial muscle tear. **B:** Ten days later the signal intensity and size of the injury are reduced as healing progresses.

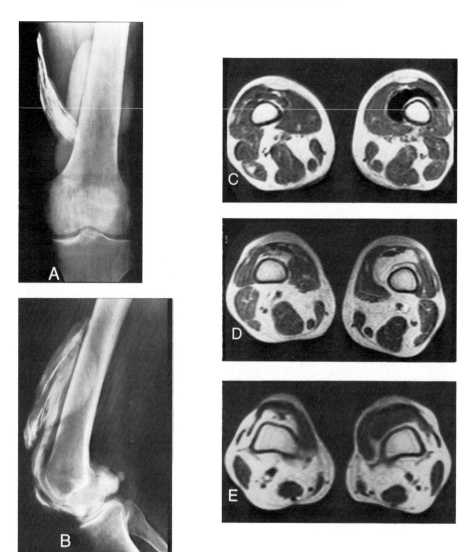

FIG. 18. Joint effusion in a patient with a large suprapatellar cyst. Anteroposterior (**A**) and lateral (**B**) radiographs following contrast injection demonstrate the abnormality. MR transaxial images show that the signal intensity of the fluid varies with the sequence used. **C:** IR (TI 400, TR 1,500): black. **D:** Spin–echo (TE 60, TR 2,000): white. **E:** Spin–echo (TE 40, TR 500): near muscle density.

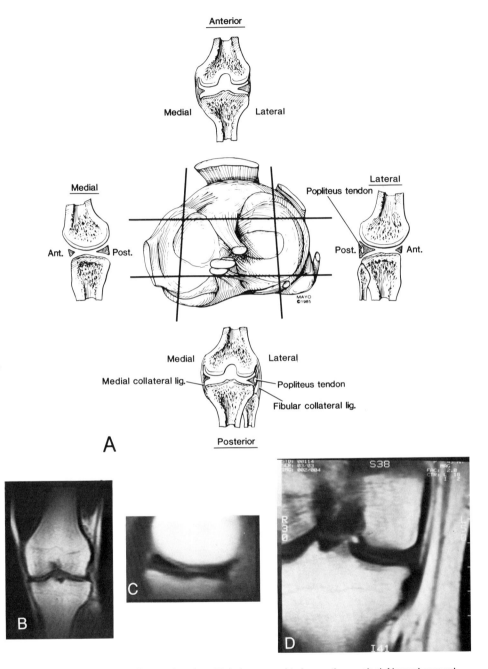

FIG. 19. A: Illustration of coronal and sagittal planes used to image the menisci. Normal coronal (**B**) and sagittal (**C**) images (TR 40, TE 500, 0.15 T) using the knee coil. **D:** Coronal surface coil image (TE 30, TR 500; 1.5 T) showing a normal medial meniscus and medial collateral ligament.

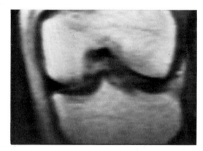

FIG. 20. Patient with previous menisectomy. The meniscus has been replaced by high signal intensity granulation tissue.

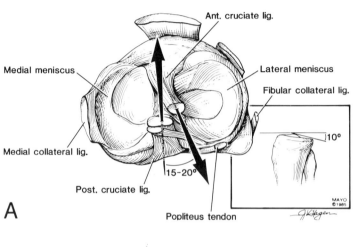

Ant. cruciate lig.

Medial meniscus

Lateral meniscus

Fibular collateral lig.

Medial collateral lig.

10°

15–20°

Post. cruciate lig.

A

Popliteus tendon

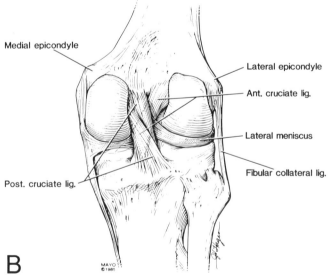

Medial epicondyle

Lateral epicondyle

Ant. cruciate lig.

Lateral meniscus

Fibular collateral lig.

Post. cruciate lig.

B

FIG. 21. Transaxial (**A**) and coronal (**B**) illustrations of the ligaments of the knee. Note the oblique course of the anterior cruciate ligament.

Therefore, if sagittal images are obtained the entire posterior cruciate can be identified in the majority of cases. We reviewed 40 four-section sagittal images of the intercondylar region and found the posterior cruciate was seen completely on one sagittal section in 37/40 (92.5%) of patients. The anterior cruciate is smaller and more difficult to study. The ligament extends obliquely from the anterior tibia, near the tibial spine, lateral to the posterior cruciate, to insert in the medial aspect of the lateral femoral condyle (Fig. 21). Therefore, in order to include the entire ligament in the image plane the knees must be externally rotated (Fig. 22). This position is difficult to maintain, and the exact angle is difficult to determine. King et al. (23) noted that the knee had to be rotated 10 to 30° in order to include the entire anterior cruciate ligament. If the knee was rotated too much, only the posterior portion of the ligament was identified. If the knee was not sufficiently rotated only the anterior portion was identified. If the knee is maintained in the neutral position our experience indicates that the

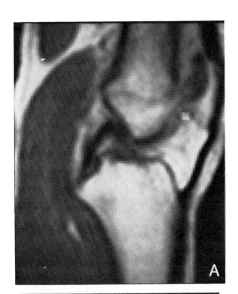

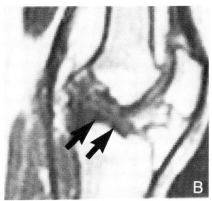

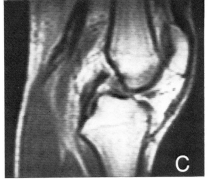

FIG. 22. Normal (**A**), torn anterior cruciate (**B**), and torn posterior cruciate ligament (**C**).

entire cruciate is seen in only 30% of patients. The anterior portion is seen in 30% and the posterior in 40% of patients. Therefore, inability to identify a portion of the ligament is not a very helpful secondary sign of ligament disruption. To further optimize visualization of the ligaments the knee should be examined in both flexion and extension. This straightens the ligaments allowing more accurate assessment. The degree of flexion is limited by coil size, but if a head coil is used, 30° of flexion can easily be obtained and extension is not a problem. The position can be maintained by using foam cushions.

Partial saturation sequences (TE 30, TR ≤ 500) can be performed quickly (short TR) and provide the best image quality. Tears in the menisci or cruciate ligaments (Fig. 22) are demonstrated as areas of increased signal intensity. Examination of both the cruciates and menisci can be very time consuming. For example, evaluation of the menisci requires at least two coronal and two sagittal multislice sequences (18 min). Both midline sagittal and rotated sagittal views are almost always needed to evaluate the cruciate ligaments (9 min). Although 27 min is not significantly longer than the time required for arthrography, one must consider that further sequences, views, and surface coil imaging may be needed. Improvements in software (off-axis field of view and oblique image planes) and coil configurations will aid in examination of the knee, but currently MR imaging is only useful in specific situations. These include muscle, extracapsular ligament, and possibly cruciate ligament injuries. MR imaging should not be used as a screening examination. Further studies are needed to determine its true role compared to arthrography and arthroscopy.

Leg

Soft tissue injuries and stress fractures of the tibia and fibula are common, especially in runners. Terms such as shinsplints, posterior and anterior compartment syndrome, and anterior and posterior tibial syndrome are frequently used to explain different pain patterns (39,43).

Stress fractures are particularly common in the untrained athlete and long distance runners. Routine radiography is not effective in early detection of stress fractures, but isotope studies allow diagnosis as early as 24 hr after the injury. Radionuclide scans are almost always by 72 hr (9,16,17,46,57). MR images may also demonstrate changes in patients with stress fractures (Fig. 23). They are seen as areas of increased signal intensity in the normally black cortical bone. These changes are most obvious on spin–echo sequences with T2-weighting (long TE and TR). There is insufficient data to determine if MR can detect stress fractures earlier, nor would this be necessarily of clinical benefit. Isotope studies are easily performed, can cover a larger area more quickly, and currently are significantly less expensive than MR techniques. They remain the technique of choice for detection of stress fractures. Radiographs and MR imaging may be useful in defining the anatomy more clearly in patients with atypical stress frac-

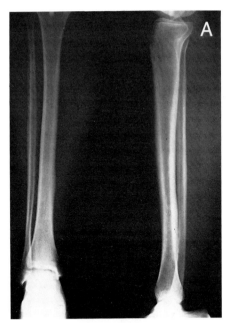
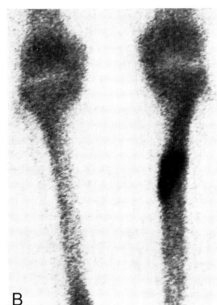
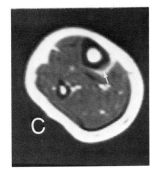

FIG. 23. Patient with suspected stress fracture. The radiographs (A) are normal. Technetium scan (B) is positive for stress
fracture. The MR image (C) also demonstrates an area of increased signal intensity in the normally black cortex (*arrow*).

tures, patients with suspected stress fractures who fail to respond to treatment,
or symptomatic patients with negative isotope scans. For example, early osteo-
genic sarcoma may mimic a stress fracture on scans and radiographs. MR imaging
generally reveals subtle neoplastic changes more readily than radiographs or
CT (9).

MR imaging is particularly useful for evaluating muscle tears, compartment
syndromes, and other post-traumatic soft tissue disorders of the leg. Strains of
the gastrocnemius and soleus muscles are particularly common: "tennis player's
leg" occurs in middle-aged players due to a second degree strain in the medial
gastrocnemius (3) (Fig. 24).

Compartment syndromes are common clinical problems. Raether and Luther
(39) stated that muscle volume may increase by 20% during exercise, partly due

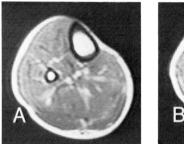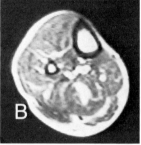

FIG. 24. Middle-aged tennis player with a partial tear of the gastrocnemius. **A:** Spin–echo (TE 40, TR 500) shows the anatomy, but the tear is only clearly demonstrated on the T2-weighted spin–echo (TE 60, TR 2,000) image (**B**).

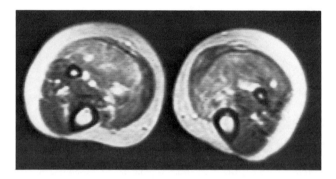

FIG. 25. Patient with suspected compartment syndrome. Transaxial image through the calf (TE 60, TR 2,000) demonstrates an infiltrative high intensity pattern with displacement of the fascia (*black*).

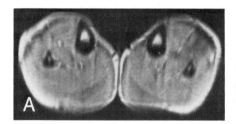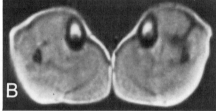

FIG. 26. Deep perineal nerve palsy on the left due to edema in the anterior compartment. Free induction decay (**A**) and IR (**B**) images.

to increased capillary filtration not compensated for by complete removal of excess fluid. Pressure can increase dramatically depending on the compliance of the fascia surrounding the muscles; tissue pressures of 40 to 60 mm Hg can lead to decreased blood flow and ischemia (55). Pressure measurements have been used in diagnosis and treatment planning, but, to date, imaging procedures

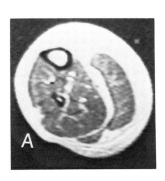 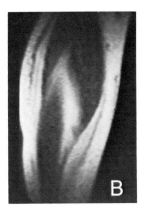

FIG. 27. Increased signal intensity on the transaxial (**A**) and sagittal (**B**) images (TE 60, TR 2,000) due to hemorrhage along the fascial plane.

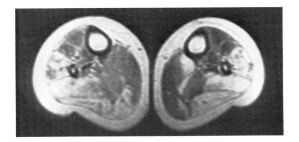

FIG. 28. Compartment syndrome with increased signal posteriorly. The muscles are distorted due to extrinsic compression by the scanner couch (patient supine).

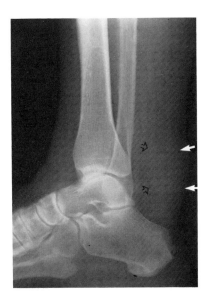

FIG. 29. Lateral view of the ankle. There is displacement of the preachilles fat (*open arrows*) and marked swelling in the region of the Achilles tendon (*white arrows*). The degree of tearing is not evident.

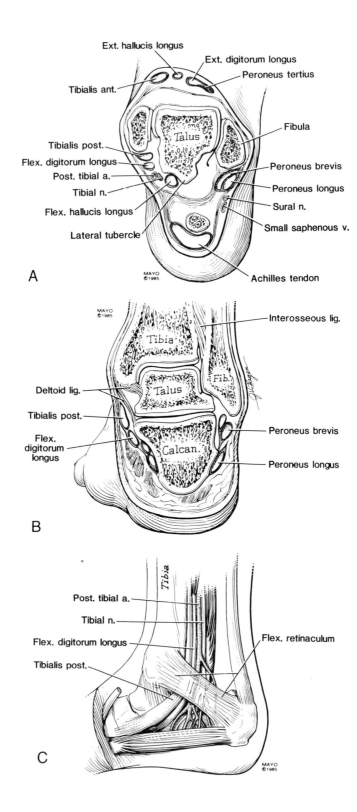

Ext. hallucis longus

Ext. digitorum longus

Peroneus tertius

Tibialis ant.

Fibula

Talus

Tibialis post.

Flex. digitorum longus

Peroneus brevis

Post. tibial a.

Peroneus longus

Tibial n.

Sural n.

Flex. hallucis longus

Small saphenous v.

Lateral tubercle

Achilles tendon

MAYO
©1985

A

Interosseous lig.

MAYO
©1985

Tibia

Fib.

Deltoid lig.

Talus

Tibialis post.

Flex. digitorum longus

Peroneus brevis

Calcan.

Peroneus longus

B

Tibia

Post. tibial a.

Tibial n.

Flex. digitorum longus

Flex. retinaculum

Tibialis post.

C

MAYO
©1985

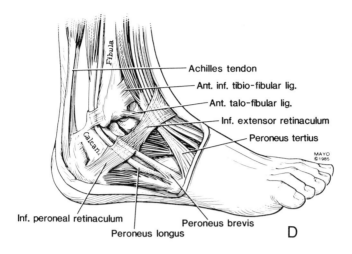

FIG. 30 (*continued.*)

have not been helpful. MR imaging can easily demonstrate changes in muscle and fascia in patients with compartment syndromes. Generally, a diffuse infiltrative high signal pattern (T2-weighted image) is present in muscle. The major fascial planes are easily identified (Figs. 25 to 28). Images demonstrate the degree and number of muscles involved, but they are not specific for etiology, as any inflammatory muscle process may give a similar appearance. The history of pain with exercise is necessary to confirm the diagnosis.

Examination of the leg is easily accomplished in knee or head coils. Usually the head coil is used, allowing comparison of both extremities (Figs. 25 to 27). Examination should include both T1- and T2-weighted sequences, and images should be performed in two planes. Most often the transaxial and coronal planes are used with the head coil. The patient should be prone if the posterior soft tissues are being studied, to avoid distortion of the tissues (Fig. 28).

Foot and Ankle

Fracture of the foot and ankle are easily assessed with routine radiographs. In certain situations tomography and isotope studies are required to detect subtle changes. Stress fractures are particularly common in the metatarsals and tarsal bones (9,16,17,22,57), where early diagnosis is established with radioisotope

FIG. 30. Illustrations of normal anatomy. **A:** Axial view demonstrating the tendons and neurovascular structures. **B:** Coronal view. **C:** Medial sagittal view. **D:** Lateral sagittal view.

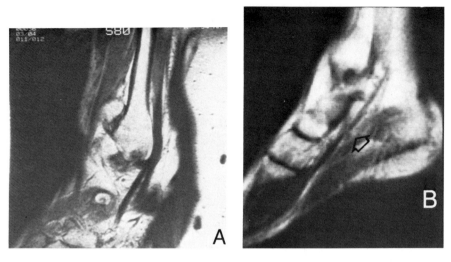

FIG. 31. A: Normal sagittal views (TE 30, TR 500; 1.5 T) of peroneal tendons. **B:** Tear in the flexor digitorum longus (0.15 T) (*arrow*).

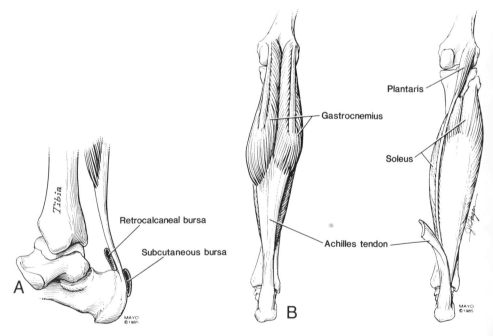

FIG. 32. Lateral (**A**) and posterior (**B**) illustration of the Achilles tendon, bursae, and calf musculature.

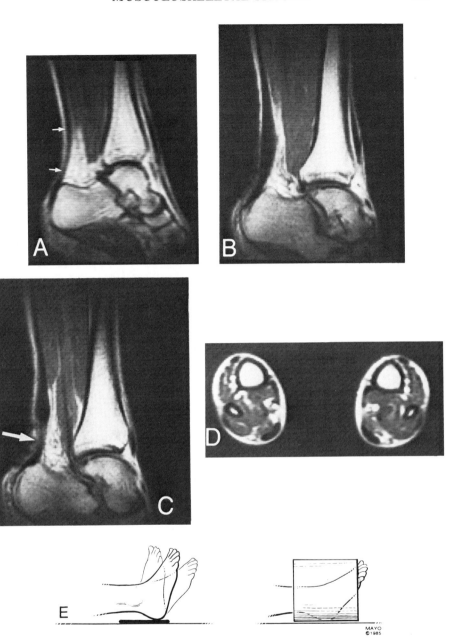

FIG. 33. A: Normal sagittal view of the Achilles tendon (*arrows*). The tendon normally appears black and has smooth margins. **B:** Inflamed thickened Achilles tendon due to chronic tendonitis. **C:** Plantar flexed foot causes deformity of the tendon, and partial volume effects from the adjacent fat mimic a tear. **D:** Axial image of the Achilles tendon in **C** was normal. Note the shape and position of the tendon. These factors must be considered to avoid false positive examinations. **E:** Illustration of flat and circular coil. Positioning can be accomplished more accurately with the flat coil.

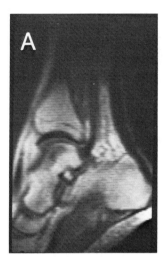

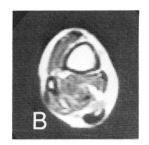

FIG. 34. Partial tear in the Achilles tendon with retrocalcaneal bursitis. **A:** Sagittal view shows slight thickening of the tendon. **B:** Axial view reveals a small tear with increased signal in the adjacent bursa.

scanning. As discussed above, MR imaging is currently of little value in evaluation of stress fractures, except in excluding other causes of positive scans (9,46).

Soft tissue injuries can be difficult to evaluate with conventional techniques, and it is in this area that MR imaging shows the most potential. Pericapsular muscle and ligament injuries are currently evaluated with stress views, arthrography, arthroscopy, and tenography (4,6,7). Ankle arthrography should be performed within 72 hr of injury for best results, but even then, a false negative rate as high as 20% has been reported in arthrographic evaluation of the calcaneofibular ligament (7). Tenography may be more accurate in evaluating the ligaments and tendons about the ankle. Most injuries of the Achilles tendon can be diagnosed clinically. Radiographic techniques may reveal secondary changes of Achilles injury, but do not allow direct assessment of the ligament (Fig. 29). Ultrasound and bursography have also provided some assistance in evaluation of this structure, but fail to provide the anatomic detail obtainable with magnetic resonance imaging.

Ankle injuries most commonly involve the lateral ligaments (7,43). The anterior talofibular ligament is involved in 67% of patients with associated involvement of the calcaneofibular ligament in about 20%. Isolated disruptions of the deltoid ligament account for only 2 to 3% of ankle ligament injuries (43). Arthrography and tenography are well suited for evaluation of the capsule and calcaneofibular ligament. Again, signs of injury are indirect and there is a significant incidence of false negative studies. MR imaging is particularly suited for evaluation of the ligaments and tendons about the ankle. Though results are preliminary, early studies of these structures are encouraging. Transaxial and sagittal planes are particularly useful in this regard (Figs. 30 and 31). Axial images localize the position of the structures, followed by thin slice sagittal images through the areas of interest. Partial saturation sequences provide the best image quality and can be performed most quickly because of the short TR (<500 msec). Examination of the articular cartilage and capsule with surface coils improves the detail and allows better evaluation of these structures.

Injuries to the Achilles tendon vary from mild tendinitis or bursitis to partial and complete thickness tears (18,45,49,50) (Figs. 32 and 33). The majority of these injuries occur in males (>80%) (47). In Smart's series (50) 44% of patients with tendon tears had received previous steroid injections, and 11% occurred in long distance runners. Pain, swelling, and weakness were the most common presenting complaints. Defects in the tendon may be palpable. Skeoch (49) reported palpable defects in 7/16 patients. Determination of the extent of the tear is important in deciding between surgical or conservative management. Ultrasound and cancaneal bursograms have been useful in certain situations, but MR examinations can be performed quickly and provide more detailed anatomic information (Fig. 33). The involved tendon is studied with multislice axial and thin slice sagittal images. The axial views are important to provide a view 90° to the sagittal and also assist in preventing over interpretation due to partial volume effects (Figs. 33C and 33D). The Achilles tendon tends to a comma shape in the axial plane and is not always perfectly midline in the sagittal plane (Fig. 33D). Thus, positioning is important to be certain that the tendon is in the sagittal plane and that the foot is not overly plantarflexed. The flat surface coil is best suited for this purpose (Fig. 33E). The latter position results in buckling of the tendon and gives the appearance of thickening (Fig. 33C). Disruptions of the tendon are demonstrated as areas of increased signal intensity, and the extent of the tear can be easily appreciated. Surrounding soft tissue changes, such as bursitis, can also be detected (Fig. 34). The response to treatment can be easily followed with MR imaging (Fig. 35).

Upper Extremities

Injuries to the upper and lower extremities occur with nearly equal frequency. Upper extremity injuries may be secondary to direct trauma (contact sports) or to ongoing stresses from throwing, swimming, and gymnastics (1,12–14,33). Skeletal injuries are usually diagnosed radiographically. Soft tissue trauma may be diagnosed by clinical exam or, if necessary, with the aid of arthrography and other imaging techniques. More recently, ultrasound has been used to evaluate rotator cuff tears. Middlestone et al. (26) detected 14/15 rotator cuff tears using ultrasound.

Evaluation of the upper limbs by MR imaging has progressed more slowly than for the lower extremities. This is largely due to difficulties in patient positioning (see T. H. Berquist, "Technical Considerations in Magnetic Resonance Imaging," *this volume*) and a lack of the needed spatial resolution to evaluate anatomy in the hand and wrist. Presently there is insufficient experience to be

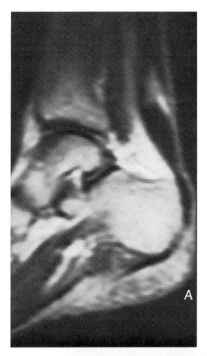

FIG. 35. Achilles tendon injury with a nearly complete tear. Initial sagittal (**A**) and axial (**B**) views demonstrate a large tear (*arrows*). Several weeks later the sagittal view shows only a small cleft like tear remains (**C**). **D:** Two months later the tendon is thickened but the tear is no longer evident. The patient was able to resume normal activities.

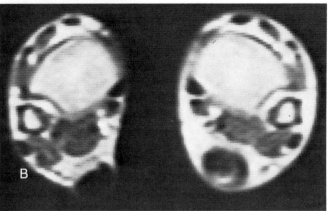

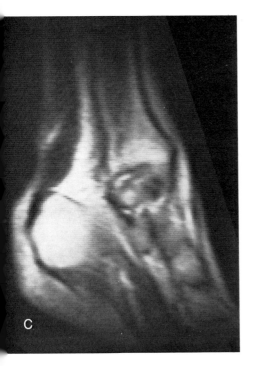
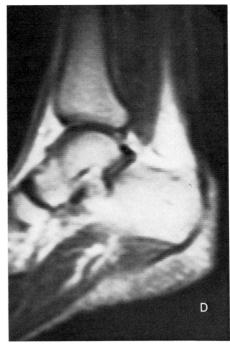

FIG. 35 (*continued.*)

TABLE 4. *Upper extremity trauma: potential uses of MR imaging*

Shoulder	Ligament injury
Rotator cuff tears	Nerve intrapment
Bursitis	Forearm
Muscle tears (biceps, pectoral)	Muscle tears
Biceps tendon injuries	Compartment syndrome
Elbow	Hand and wrist
Tendonitis	Avascular necrosis
Muscle tears	Carpal tunnel syndrome

certain what the role of MR imaging will be in evaluation of upper extremity trauma (21). Certainly, potential exists for diagnostic assistance in studies of soft tissue injury. Table 4 lists possible applications of MR imaging in the upper extremity. The development of new software and improved surface coil techniques will be of great value in this regard.

REFERENCES

1. Anderson, T. E. (1984): Shoulder injuries in the athlete. *Primary Care,* 11:129–136.
2. Andrish, J. T. (1984): Ligamentous injuries of the knee. *Primary Care,* 11:77–88.

3. Baker, B. E. (1984): Current concepts in diagnosis and treatment of musculotendinous injuries. *Med. Sci. Sports Exerc.,* 16:323–327.
4. Baker, H. L., Berquist, T. H., Kispert, D. B., Reese, D. F., Houser, W. O., Earnest, F., IV, Forbes, G. S., and May, G. R. (1985): Magnetic resonance imaging in a routine clinical setting. *Mayo Clin. Proc.,* 60:75–91.
5. Baker, C. L., Norwood, L. A., and Hughston, J. C. (1984): Acute combined posterior cruciate and posterolateral instability of the knee. *Am. J. Sports Med.,* 12:204–208.
6. Berquist, T. H. (1984): Preliminary experience in orthopedic radiology. *Magnetic Resonance Imaging,* 2:41–54.
7. Berquist, T. H. (ed.) (1985): *Imaging of Orthopedic Trauma and Surgery.* W.B. Saunders, Philadelphia.
8. Berquist, T. H. (1985): *Imaging Techniques in the Acutely Injured Patient.* Urban and Schwarzenberg, Baltimore.
9. Berquist, T. H., Cooper, K. L., and Pritchard, D. J. (1985): Stress fractures. In: *Imaging of Orthopedic Trauma and Surgery,* edited by T. H. Berquist, pp. 755–765. W.B. Saunders, Philadelphia.
10. Bowerman, J. W. (1977): *Radiology of Injury in Sports.* Appleton-Century-Crofts, New York.
11. Bryan, P. J., Butler, H. E., and LiPuma, J. P. (1984): Magnetic resonance imaging of the pelvis. *Radiol. Clin. North Am.,* 22:897–915.
12. Cofield, R. H., and Simmonet, W. T. (1984): The shoulder in sports. *Mayo Clin. Proc.,* 59:157–164.
13. Cohen, I., Lane, S., and Koning, W. (1983): Peroneal tendon dislocations: A review of the literature. *J. Foot Surg.,* 22:15–20.
14. Cooney, W. P. (1984): Sports injuries to the upper extremity. How to recognize and deal with some common problems. *Postgrad. Med.,* 76:45–50.
15. Crabtree, S. D., Bedford, A. F., and Edgar, M. A. (1981): The value of arthrography and arthroscopy in association with a sports injury clinic. A prospective and comparative study of 182 patients. *Injury,* 13:220–226.
16. Daffner, R. H. (1978): Stress fractures. *Curr. Concepts Skeletal Radiol.,* 2:221–229.
17. Devas, M. (1975): *Stress Fractures.* Churchill-Livingston, London.
18. Dickinson, P. H., Coutts, M. B., Woodward, E. P., and Handler, D. (1966): Tendoachilles bursitis. *J. Bone Joint Surg. [Am.],* 48:77–81.
19. Dorne, H. L., and Lander, P. H. (1985): Spontaneous stress fractures of the femoral neck. *A. J. R.,* 144:343–347.
20. Fornage, D. B., Rifkin, M. D., Touche, D. H., and Segal, P. M. (1984): Sonography of the patellar tendon: Preliminary observations. *A. J. R.,* 143:179–182.
21. Hinshaw, W. S., Andrew, E. R., and Bottomley, P. A. (1979): An in vivo study of the forearm by thin section NMR imaging. *Br. J. Radiol.,* 52:36–43.
22. Keats, T. E. (1984): The spectrum of musculoskeletal stress injury. *Curr. Probl. Diagn. Radiol.,* 13:7–51.
23. King, C. L., Hinkelman, R. M., Poon, P. Y., and Rubenstein, J. (1984): Magnetic resonance imaging of the normal knee. *J. Comput. Assist. Tomogr.,* 8:1147–1154.
24. McKeag, D. B. (1984): The concept of overuse: The primary care aspects of overuse syndromes in sports. *Primary Care,* 11:43–59.
25. McMaster, P. E. (1933): Tendon and muscle ruptures. *J. Bone Joint Surg. [Am.],* 15:705–722.
26. Middleton, W. D., Edelstein, G., Reinus, W. R., Melson, G. L., Totty, W. G., and Murphy, W. A. (1985): Sonographic detection of rotator cuff tears. *A. J. R.,* 144:349–353.
27. Modic, M. T., Pavlicek, W., Weinstein, W. A., Boumphrey, F., Ngo, F., Hardy, R., and Duchesneau, P. M. (1984): Magnetic resonance imaging of the vertebral disk. *Radiology,* 152:103–111.
28. Modic, M. T., Weinstein, M. A., Pavlicek, W., Boremphrey, F., Starnes, D., and Duchesneau, P. M. (1983): Magnetic resonance imaging of the cervical spine. Technical and clinical observations. *A. J. R.,* 141:1129–1136.
29. Moon, K. L., Genant, H. K., Helms, C. A., Chafetz, N. I., Crooks, L. E., and Kaufman, L. (1983): Musculoskeletal applications of nuclear magnetic resonance. *Radiology,* 147:161–171.
30. Norman, D., Mills, C. M., Brant-Zawadski, M., Yeates, A., Crooks, L. E., and Kaufman, L. (1983): Magnetic resonance imaging of the spinal cord and canal: Potentials and limitations. *A. J. R.,* 141:1147–1152.
31. Oakes, B. W. (1984): Hamstring muscle injuries. *Aust. Fam. Physician,* 13:587–591.

32. O'Donoghue, D. H. (1984): *Treatment of Injuries to Athletes. 4th Edition.* W.B. Saunders, Philadelphia.

33. Orava, S., Sorasto, A., Aalto, K., and Kvist, H. (1984): Total rupture of the pectoralis major muscle in athletes. *Int. J. Sports Med.,* 5:272–274.

34. Palmer, I. (1938): On the injuries of the ligaments of the knee joint. *Acta Chir. Scand.,* 81(Suppl. 53):11–269.

35. Paushter, D. M., and Modic, M. T. (1984): Magnetic resonance imaging of the spine. *Appl. Radiol.,* 13:61–68.

36. Pavlov, H., Hirschy, J. C., and Torg, J. (1979): Computed tomography of the cruciate ligaments. *Radiology,* 132:389–393.

37. Postacchini, F., and Ruddi, G. (1975): Subcutaneous rupture of the distal biceps brachii tendon. *J. Sports Med.,* 15:81–90.

38. Prather, J. L., Nasynowitz, M. L., Snowdy, H. A., Hughes, A. D., McCartney, W. H., and Bagg, R. J. (1977): Scintigraphic findings in stress fractures. *J. Bone Joint Surg. [Am.],* 59:869–874.

39. Raether, P. M., and Luther, L. D. (1982): Recurrent compartment syndrome in the posterior thigh. Report of a case. *Am. J. Sports Med.,* 10:40–43.

40. Rand, J. A. (1984): The role of arthroscopy in management of knee injuries in the athlete. *Mayo Clin. Proc.,* 59:77–82.

41. Reicher, M. A., Bassett, L. W., and Gold, R. H. (1985): High-resolution magnetic resonance imaging of the knee joint: Pathologic correlations. *A. J. R.,* 145:903–909.

42. Reicher, M. A., Rauschning, W., Gold, R. H., Bassett, L. W., Lufkin, R. B., and Glen, W., Jr. (1985): High-resolution magnetic resonance imaging of the knee joint: Normal anatomy. *A. J. R.,* 145:895–902.

43. Renstrom, P. (1984): Swedish research in sports traumatology. *Clin. Orthop.,* 191:144–158.

44. Ryan, A. J. (1965): Medical aspects of sports. *J. A. M. A.,* 194:643–645.

45. Santilli, G. (1979): Achilles tendonopathies and paratendonopathies. *J. Sports Med.,* 19:245–259.

46. Savoca, C. J. (1971): Stress fractures: A classification of the earliest roentgen signs. *Radiology,* 100:519–524.

47. Schneider, R., Yocavone, J., and Ghelman, G. (1985): Unsuspected sacral fractures: Detection by radionuclide bone scanning. *A. J. R.,* 144:337–341.

48. Scott, J. A., Rosenthal, D. I., and Brady, T. (1984): The evaluation of musculoskeletal diseases with magnetic resonance imaging. *Radiol. Clin. North Am.,* 22:917–924.

49. Skeoch, D. U. (1981): Spontaneous partial subcutaneous ruptures of the tendoachilles. *Am. J. Sports Med.,* 9:20–22.

50. Smart, G. W., Tauton, J. E., and Clement, D. B. (1980): Achilles tendon disorders in runners: A review. *Med. Sci. Sports Exerc.,* 12:231–243.

51. Swensen, S. J., Keller, P. J., Berquist, T. H., McLeod, R. A., and Stephens, D. H. (1985): Magnetic resonance of hemorrhage. *A. J. R.,* 145:921–927.

52. Takami, H., Takahashi, S., and Ando, M. (1983): Traumatic rupture of iliacus muscle with femoral nerve paralysis. *J. Trauma,* 23:253–254.

53. Trecco, F., DePaulis, F., Bonanni, G., Beomente-Sobel, B., Romanini, L., Passariello, R., Poppalardos, S., and Calvise, V. (1984): The use of computed tomography in the study of the cruciate ligaments of the knee. *Ital. J. Orthop. Traumatol.,* 10:109–120.

54. Turner, D. A., Prodromos, C. C., Petasnick, J. P., and Clark, J. W. (1985): Acute injury of the ligaments of the knee: Magnetic resonance evaluation. *Radiology,* 154:717–722.

55. Whitesides, T. E., Haney, T. C., and Moremoto, K. (1975): Tissue pressure measurements as a determinator for need for fasciotomy. *Clin. Orthop.,* 113:43–51.

56. Wilcox, J. R., Moniot, A. L., and Green, J. B. (1977): Bone scanning in the evaluation of exercise related stress injuries. *Radiology,* 123:699–703.

57. Wilson, E. S., and Katz, F. N. (1969): Stress fracture: An analysis of 250 consecutive cases. *Radiology,* 92:481–486.

58. Zeman, S. C. (1984): Acute knee injury. How to determine if the knee is stable. *Postgrad. Med.,* 76:38–46.

Magnetic Resonance Imaging of the Spine

Michael L. Richardson

*Department of Radiology, Harborview Medical Center, University
of Washington, Seattle, Washington 98104*

In the past 6 years, computed tomography (CT) has become the preferred modality for imaging the spine in a wide variety of disorders. However, in the past 2 years, magnetic resonance (MR) imaging has also begun to show promise as a means of accurately imaging the spine. This chapter will briefly discuss some of the technical considerations involved in spinal MR imaging. The normal anatomy of the spine will be described as seen on MR imaging, and clinical applications of MR imaging in the spine will be reviewed. Comparisons with conventional imaging techniques will also be made, and the potential and limitations of MR imaging will be discussed.

TECHNICAL CONSIDERATION

A wide variety of pulse sequences have been employed in the work-up of spinal disease with MR imaging. However, the spin–echo pulse sequence remains by far the most popular, due not only to the ease with which it can be technically implemented but also to the control it gives the operator over tissue contrast. Differences in hydrogen density and longitudinal relaxation time (T1) and transverse relaxation time (T2) of tissues form the basis for tissue characterization on MR imaging. Typical parameters for the tissues of interest in the spine are shown in Table 1 (24,25). The intrinsic contrast resolution of MR imaging between some tissues is in excess of 500%, which is far superior to the 7% typically seen with CT (11). By manipulating the imaging parameters repetition time (TR) and echo time (TE), one can increase or decrease the contrast seen between two tissues. Typical imaging parameters used in clinical MR imaging range from 300 to 3,000 msec for TR and from 30 to 120 msec for TE.

The sagittal plane is generally the most useful plane for MR imaging of the spine. Even with a short TR, one multislice scanning sequence will cover the entire cervical, thoracic, or lumbosacral spine. The axial plane is also useful but covers a much more limited segment of the spine and should probably be limited to scanning areas of special interest. Both of these planes are very convenient for viewing impingement upon the spinal canal by various processes, such as

TABLE 1. *T1 and T2 values obtained from normal tissues at 0.35 T*

Tissue	T1 (msec ± SD)	T2 (msec ± SD)	No. of samples
Muscle	541 ± 141	35 ± 6	13
Subcutaneous fat	218 ± 68	61 ± 18	12
Vertebral marrow	420 ± 112	50 ± 12	16
Nucleus pulposus	1,078 ± 396	65 ± 17	22
Anterior annulus	576 ± 338	46 ± 28	26
Posterior annulus	732 ± 266	51 ± 24	26

SD, standard deviation.

herniated discs, tumor, or osteophytes. The coronal plane is infrequently used, in part due to partial volume effects secondary to the normal spinal curvature. Special oblique views angled along the path of the nerve rootlets may be useful in some cases.

High resolution scanning and thin section slices are mandatory for accurate spinal imaging. Current imagers are now capable of slice thickness of 1.5 to 3 mm and spatial resolution of 0.9 × 0.9 mm. Some multislice imagers leave a gap between adjacent slices to minimize interslice interference. However, for spinal imaging, such a gap may cause one to miss small but important areas of pathology. Surface coil imaging shows great promise in spinal imaging. The increased signal-to-noise ratio (two to five times that of conventional head or body coils) (6) provided by the surface coil can be used to offset the increased noise incurred by using a smaller pixel size, by decreasing the slice thickness, or by reducing the amount of signal averaging to decrease the scanning time.

On the surface, pulse sequence optimization seems like a difficult problem, as there are many different MR imaging instruments to choose from, each with several different pulse sequences and potentially thousands of different combinations of TR and TE (7,12,18,22). Compounding this problem are the variations in T1, T2, and hydrogen density seen in different tissues, different patients, and different diseases. However, in practice, adequate contrast between most normal and abnormal tissues can be achieved with the simple strategy of imaging the area of interest with both a T1-weighted and a T2-weighted spin–echo sequence.

Although absolute tissue intensity can change substantially with changes in TR and TE, the relative intensity between many tissues does not change significantly over a wide range of TR/TE values (Table 2). For example, subcutaneous fat and normal marrow appear bright at most TR/TE combinations. Likewise, cortical bone, air-filled structures, fibrocartilage, and most ligaments and tendons appear very dark at most TR/TE combinations. Muscle and hyaline articular cartilage display an intermediate intensity at most TR/TE combinations. Unlike the three groups of tissues mentioned so far, a fourth group of tissues changes considerably in relative intensity with changes in TR/TE. This group generally

TABLE 2. *Signal intensity behavior of common musculoskeletal tissues*

High intensity
    Fat
    Marrow
Very low intensity
    Cortical bone
    Air
    Ligaments and tendons
    Fibrocartilage
Low to intermediate intensity
    Muscle
    Hyaline articular cartilage
Variable intensity (low intensity with T1-weighting, high intensity with T2-weighting)
    Fluid filled structures (joint effusion, thecal sac)
    Inflammatory or edematous tissue (edema)
    Neoplastic tissue
    Hematoma (intensity also varies with age of hematoma)

has long T1 (700 to 2,000 msec) and T2 (60 to 200 msec) relaxation times and consists of fluid-filled structures (e.g., thecal sac), edematous tissue, and most tumors. Controversy exists as to why tumors have such elevated T1 times, but increased tissue water seems to play a role (3,9,26). With a T1-weighted sequence (e.g., TR/TE of 500/30 msec), tissue in this fourth group generally appears low in intensity and becomes very bright on T2-weighted sequences (e.g., TR/TE of 2,000/60 msec). One can easily exploit this behavior in choosing a pulse sequence protocol. For example, in a patient with metastatic carcinoma involving the spine, one would like to maximize contrast between tumor and the normal background tissues of that area, i.e., fat, marrow, and cerebrospinal fluid (CSF). With a T1-weighted sequence, fat and marrow will be bright, whereas tumors and CSF will be relatively dark (Fig. 1). With a more T2-weighted sequence, fat and marrow will remain bright, whereas tumor and CSF become brighter than before.

In general, the more widely one separates the TR/TE values in these T1- and T2-weighted sequences, the better the contrast that is achieved between tumor and normal tissue. However, this must be balanced against the practical considerations of imaging time and patient comfort. Multiecho pulse sequences have been implemented on many scanners. These sequences allow the acquisition of images at multiple values of TE without increasing the total scanning time.

A typical protocol for spinal imaging in our institution usually consists of three sequences. A T1-weighted (e.g., TR/TE of 500/30 msec) sagittal series of images is obtained. This is followed by a T2-weighted (e.g., TR/TE of 2,000/60 msec) sagittal series. This is in turn followed by an axial series directed through the area of greatest interest. This axial sequence is often performed with an intermediate value of TR and TE (e.g., TR/TE of 1,600/300 msec). The T1-weighted sagittal sequence shows good contrast between marrow or epidural fat

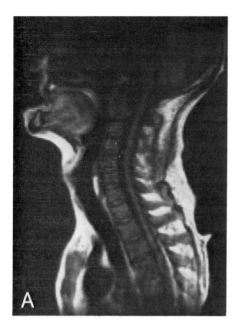 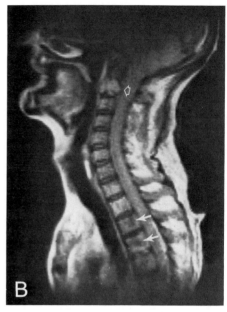

FIG. 1. Elderly male with mixed lytic and blastic metastases to the cervical spine from prostatic carcinoma. **A:** T1-weighted image (TR/TE of 500/28 msec, 0.35 T). Note the low intensity of all vertebral bodies due to diffuse infiltration of the marrow by tumor. A focal lytic metastasis is noted in the base of C2. **B:** T2-weighted image (TR/TE of 1,500/56 msec). The marrow has increased in intensity significantly. The focal metastasis at C2 has also increased in intensity, and its posterior margin is now more clearly seen where it indents the thecal sac (*open arrow*). Focal blastic lesions are seen in the vertebral bodies of T3 and T4 (*solid arrows*). These lesions did not increase in intensity with T2-weighting.

and CSF, tumor, and inflammatory tissue. The T2-weighted sequence shows better contrast between tumor and CSF, normal disc versus degenerated disc, or herniated disc versus CSF. Besides yielding extra views of the area of interest, the axial series is often useful for delineating the extent of processes such as inflammatory disease or tumor, as the plane is perpendicular to most of the important tissue planes in the paraspinal area. The preceding combination of spin–echo pulse sequences yields images with adequate contrast between normal spinal tissues and most pathological processes with both a 0.15 and a 0.35 T system.

NORMAL ANATOMY

Normal spinal anatomy is demonstrated quite nicely by MR imaging (Fig. 2). The vertebral bodies have a high signal intensity due to the marrow fat and are outlined by a thin dark line which represents the cortical bone and end-plates.

The intervertebral discs display a relatively bright signal and are bounded anteriorly and posteriorly by a thin zone of low intensity, which probably represents the Sharpey's fibers (outer fibers of the annulus). No discrete boundary is seen between the nucleus pulposus and the inner fibers of the annulus, although contrast between these areas increases with T2-weighted images (19,25). A thin linear area of low intensity is seen in the center of most discs after the third decade (Fig. 3) and has been termed the intranuclear cleft (1). This cleft is seen as part of the normal aging process and probably represents an area of progressive invagination of fibrous tissue into the nuclear material. This cleft is a very constant finding on high quality sagittal MR images of the spine after the third decade. If absent in a disc of such a patient, one should consider the possibility of disc infection at that level (13). A thin layer of high intensity epidural fat is often seen along the posterior border of the vertebral bodies. This epidural fat is also seen extending into the neural foramina bilaterally, where it surrounds the nerve rootlets. The interspinous ligaments, the ligamenta flava, and the margins of the facet joints appear as areas of very low intensity in their expected anatomic locations. The anterior and posterior ligaments are closely applied to the vertebral bodies and blend into the outer annular fibers of the discs. These ligaments are not seen as separate structures.

CLINICAL APPLICATIONS

Degenerative Disease

With degenerative disc disease, many of the same findings seen on plain radiographs are also noted on MR scans, such as intervertebral disc space narrowing and marginal osteophytosis (Fig. 4). A finding unique to MR imaging is the decreased intensity seen on T2-weighted images in degenerated disc material when compared to normal disc material (Fig. 5). This is presumably due to decreased hydration in the degenerated disc.

Herniated disc material can be well seen with MR imaging, especially on sagittal images. Figure 6 shows a large herniated disc at L5–S1. Transaxial MR imaging can also demonstrate a herniated disc and is probably more likely to demonstrate a lateral disc herniation than a sagittal series. Although not all degenerated discs do not herniate, almost all herniated discs do degenerate (15). Thus a sagittal T2-weighted study can provide a rapid screening examination for the presence of disc disease.

High resolution CT is still superior to MR imaging in the evaluation of subtle bony changes, osteophytes, or small disc calcifications. However, with surface coil technology, the spatial resolution of MR imaging is nearly equivalent to that of state of the art CT scanners (5) and provides an examination that is equivalent to CT and/or myelography (Fig. 7). In a prospective study of 60 patients, Modic et al. compared surface coil MR to CT and myelography (14).

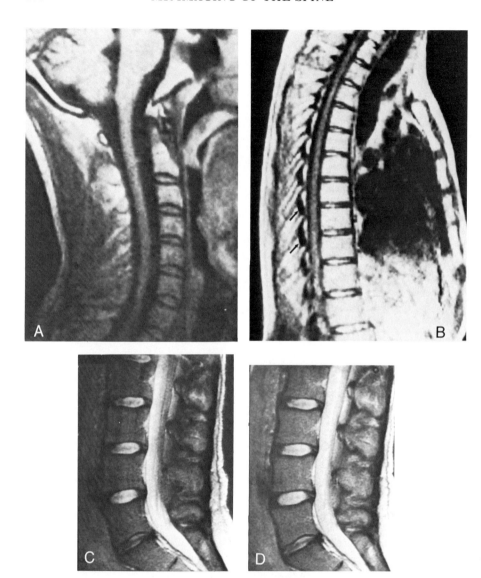

FIG. 2. Normal anatomy. **A:** Sagittal T1-weighted (TR/TE of 600/30 msec, 0.15 T) image of the normal cervical spine. With this sequence, the cord is shown nicely against the darker CSF. The craniovertebral junction and prevertebral soft tissues are also well demonstrated. **B:** T1-weighted image of a normal thoracic spine, showing the intermediate intensity of the spinal cord outlined by darker CSF. The low intensity ligamenta flava (*arrows*) are seen extending between the spinous processes. **C, D:** Sagittal surface coil images (1.5 T) of the lumbar spine with TR 2,000, and TE of 50 (**C**) and 100 (**D**). There is a thin layer of epidural fat posterior to the bodies. Note the increase in signal intensity of the discs, spinal fluid, and vertebrae as the TE is increased. There are early degenerative changes in the L4 and lumbosacral discs. **E:** Sagittal T1-weighted (TR/TE of 600/40, 0.15 T) image of a normal lumbar spine showing multiple Schmorl's nodes.

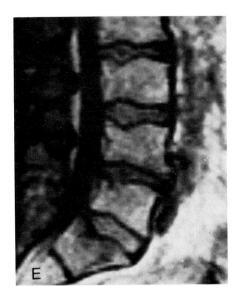

FIG. 2. (*continued.*)

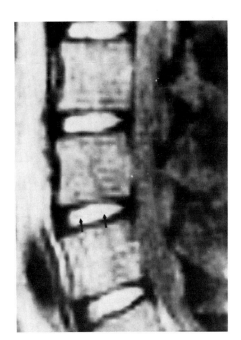

FIG. 3. T2-weighted sagittal image (TR/TE of 2,000/56 msec, 0.35 T) of the lumbar spine in a 26 year old male. Note the intranuclear clefts at several disc levels (*arrows*).

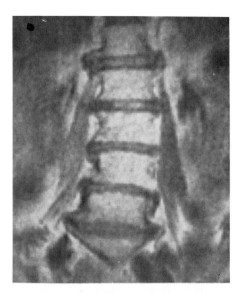

FIG. 4. Coronal T1-weighted image (TR/TE of 600/40 msec, 0.15 T) of the lumbar spine of an 82 year old male with degenerative disc disease of the lumbar spine. Decreased intervertebral disc height and marginal osteophytosis are noted at several levels.

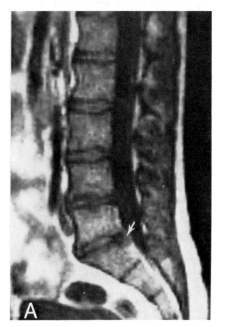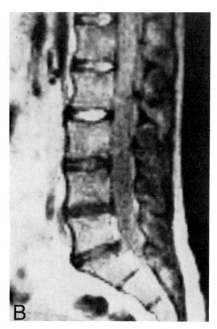

FIG. 5. Thirty-one year old male with sciatica. **A:** T1-weighted sagittal image (TR/TE of 500/28 msec, 0.35 T) shows narrowed disc spaces at L4–5 and L5–S1, as well as a posteriorly herniated disc at L5–S1 (*arrow*). **B:** T2-weighted image (TR/TE of 1,500/56 msec) shows increased signal intensity in the normal disc at L2–3. The discs at L3–4, L4–5, and L5–S1 remain low in intensity, consistent with degenerative disc disease. The herniated disc is much better seen on this sequence and has completely effaced the adjacent epidural fat.

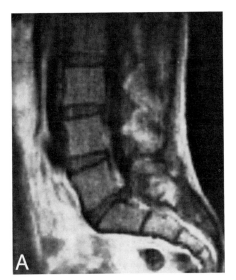 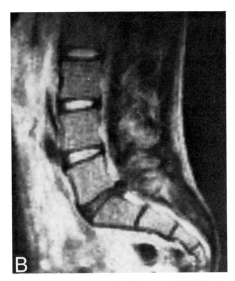

FIG. 6. Twenty-six year old male with sciatica. **A:** T1-weighted sagittal image (TR/TE of 500/28 msec, 0.35 T) of the lumbar spine shows a large herniated disc at L5–S1. Note that this disc is isointense with the other discs at this sequence. **B:** T2-weighted image (TR/TE of 2,000/ 56 msec) shows decreased intensity of the L5–S1 disc, and normal intensity in the other discs, which are normal.

At 62 operated levels, there was an 83% agreement between surgery and both MR imaging and CT, while myelography agreed with surgery in 72%. When MR imaging and CT were used jointly, the agreement with surgery rose to 91%. When CT and myelography were used jointly, they agreed with surgery in 88% of the levels. When the three modalities were compared independent of the

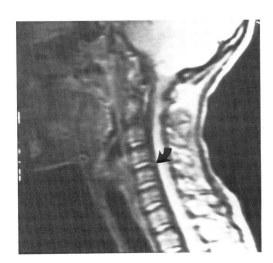

FIG. 7. Surface coil image (1.5 T) of the cervical spine with a herniated disc at C4 (*arrow*).

surgically operated levels, agreement was seen between MR imaging and CT in all patients at 151 levels and between MR imaging and myelography in 218 levels.

The diagnosis and grading of spinal stenosis can be accomplished by MR imaging. The presence of large osteophytes, ligamentum flavum hypertrophy, and disc bulging can usually be seen quite well with MR imaging (Fig. 8). The dimensions of the spinal canal, lateral recesses, and neural foramina can be easily measured. The size of the thecal sac and the presence of effacement by external structures can be assessed. While high-resolution CT is currently superior to MR imaging in the evaluation of small bony changes or calcification, surface coil MR imaging is improving rapidly and may soon equal or surpass CT in this area.

Trauma

MR imaging has not yet been extensively evaluated in the work-up of spinal trauma (see T. H. Berquist, R. L. Ehman, J. A. Rand, and A. Scott, *this volume*). Although a wide variety of monitoring devices can now be used within an imager, there are still potential problems in examining patients with large ferromagnetic stabilizing devices. This problem could be resolved by using small nonferromagnetic stabilizing devices and minimized by resorting to a low field imager.

Because of its ability to directly demonstrate the spinal cord and canal, hematoma, and fracture fragments in multiple planes (see Fig. 9) without contrast agents and without moving a critically injured patient, MR imaging has great potential in evaluating the acutely traumatized spine. For example, if one could

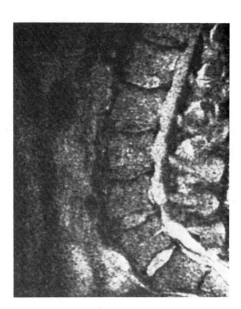

FIG. 8. Sagittal MR image (TE 100, TR 2,000) of the lumbar spine showing bulging of the lower disc annuli and spinal canal compression due to the annular bulging and hypertrophy of the ligamentum flavum.

reliably distinguish patients with spinal shock without cord transection from those with partial or complete transection, this could be of great therapeutic and prognostic significance.

Subacute fractures of the spine show increased intensity on both T1- and T2-weighted images, possibly secondary to the presence of hemorrhage about the fracture zone. Chronic compression fractures have a variable appearance (Fig. 9), depending upon their age, the degree of callus formation and fragment impaction, and perhaps other factors as well.

Infection

MR imaging is very sensitive at demonstrating inflammatory disease of the musculoskeletal system, and in the spine, it has been shown to be as sensitive and accurate as radionuclide studies. Although many of the MR imaging findings of spinal infection are similar to those of other entities, such as tumor or degenerative disease, the pattern of disease involvement in spinal infection is characteristic enough that these other entities can often be excluded with confidence. It should be stressed that MR imaging is not appropriate as a whole body screening test for infection. Rather, it should be used as a directed examination of a certain body part, based upon clinical information and the results of other tests.

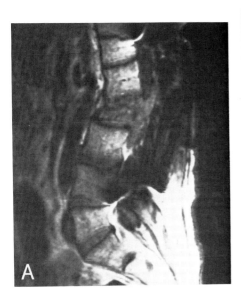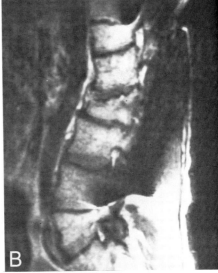

FIG. 9. Compression fracture of L2: Sagittal views of the lumbar spine with TE 30, TR 500 (**A**) and TE 50, TR 2,000 (**B**) show compression of L2 with kyphotic angulation. The cord is not well seen due to artifact from the recently placed Harrington rods. Except for the fracture (low intensity) the signal intensity of the body is only minimally different from the normal vertebrae with long TE, TR (**B**).

As one might expect, the edema and increased water content associated with inflammation appears as an area of low intensity on T1-weighted images and as a high intensity area on T2-weighted images, especially along the end-plates (Fig. 10). These intensity changes do not rule out other diseases. However, their pattern of occurrence and other associated findings make the diagnosis of infection much more certain. These associated findings include loss of disc height, especially if rapid, loss of the discrete border between the vertebral endplate and the disc, and abnormal configuration or absence of the intranuclear cleft (13).

In a recent study of 37 patients clinically suspected of vertebral osteomyelitis (13), MR imaging was found to have a sensitivity of 96%, a specificity of 93%, and an accuracy of 94%. This compared well with the combined gallium/technetium scans, which had a sensitivity of 90%, a specificity of 100%, and an accuracy of 94%. However, MR imaging was found to be more accurate anatomically than the radionuclide studies and offered significant anatomic information regarding the adjacent thecal sac and neural structures. Involvement of the vertebral bodies, discs, and paravertebral region were more apparent on MR, even when compared to single photon emission computed tomography (SPECT). MR imaging can demonstrate the findings of osteomyelitis as early as a gallium study can, and the results of an MR imaging examination are usually available within 30 to 45 min, compared to the hours or days necessary to perform a technetium or gallium study, respectively.

Although degenerative disc disease also leads to disc space narrowing, such discs remain low in intensity with a T2-weighted sequence. Whereas metastatic disease very commonly affects the vertebral bodies, it is quite uncommon for it to involve the intervertebral discs (16,21).

The relationship between antibiotic therapy and MR imaging findings has not

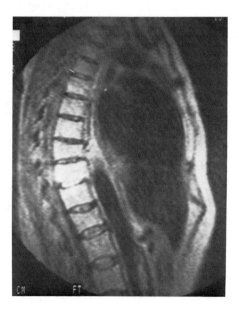

FIG. 10. Sagittal image of the thoracic spine showing increased signal intensity in the disc and body due to infection (TE 60, TR 2,000).

yet been completely evaluated. Previous antibiotic therapy may alter the MR imaging findings somewhat, but they are not obscured in the early stages as with gallium scanning (13). However, MR imaging abnormalities may linger after the infection has healed and the gallium scan has returned to normal. Therefore, it would appear that although MR imaging can be very useful in the work-up of vertebral infection, conventional radionuclide scintigraphy still may have a role in the follow-up of treatment.

Neoplasms

Primary or metastatic neoplasms of the spine are well seen against the bright marrow background. In general, blastic metastases present as an area of low signal intensity regardless of the TR/TE combination used (Fig. 1). Primary tumors that produce a sclerotic reaction, such as osteoid osteoma, or that produce tumor bone, such as osteosarcoma (Fig. 11), may demonstrate similar behavior. On the other hand, lytic metastases, diffuse marrow infiltration by tumor, and primary tumors with a large soft tissue component appear as areas of decreased signal intensity on T1-weighted images and increased signal intensity on T2-

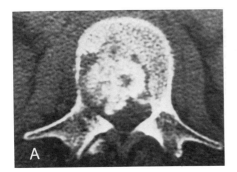
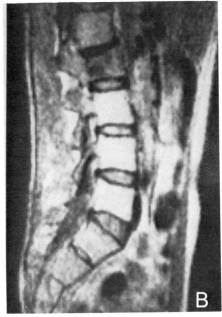

FIG. 11. Nineteen year old male with metastatic osteosarcoma to the L2 vertebral body. **A:** CT scan through L2 shows a lytic lesion involving the vertebral body with a pathological fracture and tumor bone formation bulging back into the spinal canal. **B:** Right parasagittal T1-weighted image (TR/TE of 600/40 msec, 0.15 T) of the lumbar spine shows an area of low intensity in the vertebral body of L2. The vertebral body is decreased in height, consistent with a fracture. Destruction of the right pedicle of L2 and obliteration of most of the right L2–3 neural foramen is also noted.

weighted images. Marrow infiltration is best shown with a T1-weighted image, whereas impingement upon adjacent structures, such as the spinal cord, may be best shown on more T2-weighted images (Fig. 1). Because of its limited scanning field, MR imaging is not suitable for screening the entire body for metastatic disease. However, when directed by other tests or clinical information, it may be extremely useful in demonstrating tumor location, extent, and its relation to vital structures.

MR has not been shown to be generally useful for the histological grading of tumors, other than for fatty tumors such as lipomas or low-grade liposarcomas or of fluid-filled lesions, such as aneurysmal bone cysts (8), which may be suspected by the presence of a fluid-fluid level or by the presence of an extremely long T1 or T2 relaxation time.

Other Infiltrative Diseases of Marrow

The relative distribution of red (hematopoietic) versus yellow (fatty) marrow changes dramatically with age, stress, or disease (10). Diseases such as leukemia, lymphoma, Gaucher's disease, or anemias such as aplastic anemia or sickle thalassemia can have profound effects on the normally bright marrow signal seen in the spine.

Very close correlation has been shown between the extent of marrow intensity changes on MR imaging and the histological grade of marrow involvement estimated by marrow biopsy (Fig. 12). In a recent study of 40 adults with leukemia or lymphoma (17), 17 of 18 patients with abnormal MR imaging studies were shown to have hypercellular marrow on biopsy. Of the remaining 22 patients with normal MR imaging studies, all 22 were found to have normal or hypocellular marrow on biopsy. The ability to noninvasively predict the extent of marrow involvement has important therapeutic ramifications, as decisions on chemotherapy or radiation therapy are often based on the degree of marrow infiltration. In patients treated for their disease by bone marrow transplantation, the dosage and timing of immunosuppressive drugs may depend upon changes in marrow cellularity.

Not all marrow-based disorders cause diffuse marrow replacement. Lymphoma is known for its tendency to form focal nodules of tumor. MR imaging may detect such focal involvement of the marrow prior to the development of more diffuse disease before even the bone scan becomes positive. However, the sensitivity and specificity of MR imaging for evaluating focal disease in this fashion is currently unknown.

Postoperative Changes

Following surgical discectomy, a decreased intervertebral disc space is usually noted on MR imaging. Surgical discectomy or spinal fusion may also be followed by intensity changes (low intensity on T1-weighted images and higher intensity on T2-weighted images) in the vertebral bodies and posterior soft tissues for up

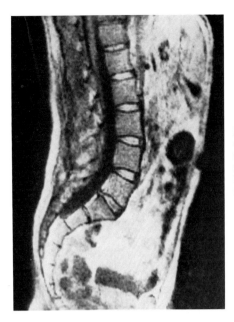

FIG. 12. Forty-four year old male with hairy-cell leukemia. This sagittal T1-weighted image (TR/TE of 600/40 msec, 0.15 T) shows a diminished signal intensity throughout the lumbosacral spine consistent with diffuse infiltration by leukemic cells.

to 6 to 12 months (Fig. 13). Anecdotal evidence suggests that MR imaging may be able to differentiate postoperative fibrosis from recurrent disc disease or retained disc fragments in some patients (2). However, the intensity of postoperative fibrosis may vary greatly and may be isointense with disc material in some cases.

Within 6 to 8 weeks following chemonucleolysis of a disc, narrowing of the disc space, decreased intensity of the disc material, and, frequently, retraction

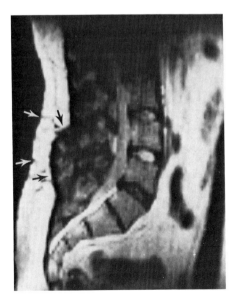

FIG. 13. Thirty-three year old male with a T2-weighted sagittal image (TR/TE of 2,000/56 msec, 0.35 T) performed 10 months after a discectomy at L5–S1 for a herniated nucleus pulposus. Note the decreased height and intensity of the intervertebral disc space compared to the normal disc at L4–5. Also note the postoperative changes in the posterior paraspinal soft tissue (*arrows*).

of herniated disc material are noted (Fig. 14). On very T2-weighted images, increased intensity may be seen adjacent to the end-plates in these patients (Fig. 15).

Postradiation Changes

An early study of 4 patients treated with 4,000 to 5,790 rads showed well-defined areas of increased signal intensity in the vertebral bodies which corresponded closely to treatment portals (20) (Fig. 16). This was best seen in the midsagittal plane on T1-weighted sequences and was felt to represent replacement of the normal cellular elements of marrow with fatty tissue. Since recurrent tumor typically appears as areas of low intensity on a T1-weighted sequence, tumor involvement was easily differentiated from radiation changes.

CONTRAST AGENTS

The role of intravenous paramagnetic MR contrast agents in spinal imaging is not yet known, and little work has been done in this field. One early study (27) showed improvement in the contrast between tumor and normal tissue following gadolinium diethylenetriamine pentacetic acid (Gd-DTPA) administration. Perhaps these agents will someday help to resolve some of the currently difficult diagnostic problems in MR imaging of the spine, such as distinguishing postoperative scarring from recurrent or retained disc.

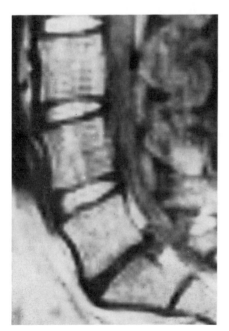

FIG. 14. The patient in Fig. 6 underwent injection of chymopapain into the disc at L5–S1 soon after that image was obtained. This image (TR/TE of 2,000/28 msec, 0.35 T) was obtained approximately 6 weeks following the injection. Note the marked decrease in both disc height and intensity since the prior scan. Although the herniated disc shows little or no retraction since the prior exam, the patient experienced dramatic relief of symptoms.

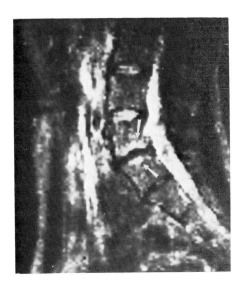

FIG. 15. A strongly T2-weighted sagittal image (TR/TE of 3,000/120 msec, 0.35 T) of another patient's lumbosacral spine following chemopapain injection at L5–S1. At this sequence, the marrow signal is quite dark, but CSF is very bright. Also note the increased signal intensity along the end-plates on either side of the L5–S1 disc space (*arrows*).

OTHER PULSE SEQUENCES

This discussion has so far dealt almost exclusively with the spin–echo pulse sequence. However, other sequences, such as inversion recovery (IR) or partial saturation recovery may be useful in certain circumstances.

The Dixon sequence, which allows one to create separate images for fat and

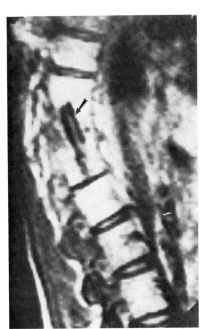

FIG. 16. T1-weighted parasagittal image (TR/TE of 600/40 msec, 0.15 T) of the thoracolumbar spine of a young patient treated for Ewing's sarcoma of the T11 vertebral body. This lesion was treated with surgery, a fibular graft (*arrow*), and local radiation therapy. Note the relative increase in signal intensity in the T10, T12, and L1 vertebral bodies, which were within the radiation portal.

water (4) (Fig. 17), may prove useful in the spine in disorders such as osteoporosis. The vertebral bodies are composed of predominantly trabecular bone, compared to tubular bones such as the radius, which may contain only 5 to 25% trabecular bone. This trabecular bone is not only much more metabolically active than cortical bone but also contains proportionally much more marrow than tubular bones. One of the current problems with spinal densitometry by CT or dual photon absorptiometry has been the increased amount of fatty yellow marrow seen in the vertebral bodies of many elderly patients. This increased fat content lowers the average attenuation value of the vertebral spongiosa and may result in an underestimation of approximately 21 to 31 mg/cm^3 in the CT spinal mineral measurement (23). With the use of a modified Dixon sequence or with the development of spatially localized proton spectroscopy, it may be possible to provide an independent and noninvasive measure of the fat content of vertebral bodies, which can be used to correct the mineral readings found by other modalities.

CONCLUSIONS

CT has been the procedure of choice for disc disease, trauma, and many other disorders of the spine for several years. However, it is clear that MR imaging has the potential to equal or surpass the utility of CT in most spinal imaging. Growing evidence suggests that MR imaging can already equal or surpass conventional studies in the management of disc disease, vertebral osteomyelitis, spinal neoplasia, and disease recurrence following radiation therapy to the spine.

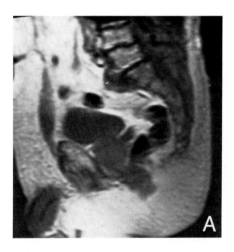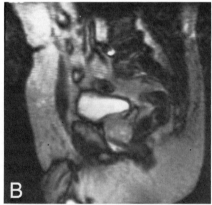

FIG. 17. Dixon sequence image of spine of the lumbosacral spine (TE 25, TR 1,000). **A:** The in-phase sagittal image demonstrates normal marrow signal with degenerative disc disease. **B:** Phase contrast image shows marked reduction in signal of the marrow due to balance of fat and water protons. There is increased signal anterior to L5–S1 due to inflammation and increased water. There are also inflammatory changes in the prostate.

Further studies will better define the role of MR imaging, CT, and radionuclide scintigraphy in the diagnosis of spinal disease.

REFERENCES

1. Aguila, L. A., Piraino, D. W., Modic, M. T., et al. (1985): The intranuclear cleft of the intervertebral disc: Magnetic resonance imaging. *Radiology,* 155:155–158.
2. Chafetz, N. I., Genant, H. K., Moon, K. L., Helms, C. A., and Morris, J. M. (1983): Recognition of lumbar disk herniation with NMR. *A. J. R.,* 141:1153–1156.
3. Damadian, R. (1971): Tumor detection by nuclear magnetic resonance. *Science,* 171:1151–1153.
4. Dixon, W. T. (1984): Simple proton spectroscopic imaging. *Radiology,* 153:189–194.
5. Edelman, R. R., Shoukimas, G. M., Stark, D. D., et al. (1985): High-resolution surface coil imaging of lumbar disk disease. *A. J. N. R.,* 6:479–485.
6. Fisher, M. R., Barker, B., Amparo, E. G., et al. (1985): MR imaging using specialized coils. *Radiology,* 157:443–447.
7. Hendrick, R. E., Nelson, T. R., and Hendee, W. R. (1984): Optimizing tissue contrast in magnetic resonance imaging. *Magnetic Resonance Imaging,* 2:113–204.
8. Hudson, T. M., Hamlin, D. J., and Fitzsimmons, J. R. (1985): Magnetic resonance imaging of fluid levels in an aneurysmal bone cyst and in anticoagulated human blood. *Skeletal Radiol.,* 13:267–270.
9. Kiricuta, I., and Simplaceanu, V. (1975): Tissue water content and nuclear magnetic resonance in normal and tumor tissues. *Cancer Res.,* 35:1164–1167.
10. Kricun, M. E. (1985): Red-yellow marrow conversion: Its effect on the location of some solitary bone lesions. *Skeletal Radiol.,* 14:10–19.
11. Margulis, A. R., Crooks, L. E., and Kaufman, L. (1984): Present clinical status of magnetic resonance imaging. In: *Biomedical Magnetic Resonance,* edited by T. L. James and A. R. Margulis, pp. 301–308. University of California, San Francisco.
12. Mitchell, M. R., Conturo, T. E., Gruber, T. H., and Jones, J. P. (1984): Two computer models for selection of optimal magnetic resonance imaging (MRI) pulse sequence timing. *Invest. Radiol.,* 19:350–360.
13. Modic, M. T., Feiglin, D. H., Piraino, D. W., et al. (1985): Vertebral osteomyelitis: Assessments using MR. *Radiology,* 157:157–166.
14. Modic, M. T., Masaryk, T. J., Boumphrey, F., et al. (1985): A prospective comparison of surface coil MRI, CT and myelography in the diagnosis of lumbar herniated disk disease and canal stenosis. *Ann. Meet. Am. Roentgen Ray Soc., Boston, 1985.*
15. Modic, M. T., Weinstein, M. A., Pavlicek, W., et al. (1984): Magnetic resonance imaging of intervertebral disc disease—clinical and pulse sequence considerations. *Radiology,* 152:103–111.
16. Norman, A., and Kambolis, C. P. (1964): Tumors of the spine and their relationship to the intervertebral disc. *A. J. R.,* 92:1270–1274.
17. Olson, D. O., Shields, A. F., Schewich, C. J., Porter, B. A., and Moss, A. A. (1985): Magnetic resonance imaging of the bone marrow in patients with leukemia, aplastic anemia and lymphoma. *Ann. Meet. Soc. Mag. Res. Med., London, Aug., 1985.*
18. Ortendahl, D. A., Hylton, N., Kaufman, L., et al. (1984): Analytical tools for magnetic resonance imaging. *Radiology,* 153:479–488.
19. Pech, P. E., and Haughton, V. M. (1985): Lumbar intervertebral disc: Correlated MR and anatomic study. *Radiology,* 156:699–701.
20. Ramsey, R. G., and Zacharias, C. E. (1985): MRI imaging of the spine after radiation therapy: Easily recognizable effects. *A. J. R.,* 144:1131–1135.
21. Resnick, D., and Niwayama, G. (1978): Intervertebral disc abnormalities associated with vertebral metastases: Observations in patients and cadavers with prostate cancer. *Invest. Radiol.,* 13:182–190.
22. Richardson, M. L., Amparo, E. G., Gillespy, T., III, Helms, C. A., Demas, B. E., and Genant, H. K. (1985): Theoretical considerations for optimizing intensity differences between primary musculoskeletal tumors and normal tissue with spin-echo magnetic resonance imaging. *Invest. Radiol.,* 20:492–497.

23. Richardson, M. L., Genant, H. K., Cann, C. E., et al. (1985): Assessment of metabolic bone diseases by quantitative computed tomography. *Clin. Orthop.,* 185:224–238.
24. Richardson, M. L., Genant, H. K., Helms, C. A., et al. (1985): Magnetic resonance imaging of the musculoskeletal system. *Orthop. Clin. North Am.,* 16:569–587.
25. Richardson, M. L., Gillespy, T., III, Horton, K., et al. (1984): Optimization of pulse sequences for spin-echo magnetic resonance imaging of intervertebral disc disease. *Radiology,* 153(P):202.
26. Saryan, L. A., Hollis, D. P., Economou, J. S., and Eggleston, J. C. (1974): Nuclear magnetic resonance studies of cancer. IV. Correlation of water content with tissue relaxation times. *J. N. C. I.,* 52:599–602.
27. Worthington, B. S., Steiner, R. E., Jelliffe, A. M., Mulholland, R. C., Young, I., and Gyngell, M. (1984): The role of MR imaging in the evaluation of intrinsic bone tumors. *Radiology,* 153(P):115.

Miscellaneous Conditions and Future Potential

Thomas H. Berquist, Richard L. Ehman,
*Michael L. Richardson, †Clyde A. Helms,
and §Harry K. Genant

*Mayo Medical School, and Department of Diagnostic Radiology, Mayo Clinic,
Rochester, Minnesota 55905; *Department of Radiology, Harborview Medical Center,
University of Washington, Seattle, Washington 98104; †Department of Radiology,
University of California School of Medicine, San Francisco, California 94143
§Department of Radiology, Medicine, and Orthopedic Surgery, University of
California School of Medicine, San Francisco, California 94143*

The previous chapters have discussed basic principles and the types of musculoskeletal pathology that have been most extensively studied with magnetic resonance (MR) techniques. MR has also demonstrated significant potential in other areas, but experience is more limited. Despite this limited experience, the potential application of MR imaging in these areas deserves mention.

OSTEONECROSIS

Osteonecrosis is a general term applied to conditions resulting in necrosis of bone and marrow elements. The term avascular necrosis is most commonly applied when the epiphyses or subchondral bone is involved. Osteonecrosis of the metaphyseal or diaphyseal bone is commonly referred to as a bone infarct (24).

Bone necrosis occurs when flow is disrupted by thrombosis, external compression, vessel wall disease, or traumatic disruption of vessels. There are numerous causes of osteonecrosis which may involve many areas of the skeleton (24). Table 1 summarizes the common etiological factors and locations of osteonecrosis.

Early diagnosis and selection of the most suitable therapy has been particularly challenging in patients with avascular necrosis (AVN) of the hip. Initial clinical symptoms may be minimal or misleading. Treatment is controversial, but many surgeons feel core decompression is effective if the diagnosis can be established early. Reports have demonstrated a gradual decrease in flow to the femoral head when systemic corticosteroids are used. Flow gradually returned to normal fol-

TABLE 1. *Osteonecrosis: etiology and locations*

Common sites of involvement	Etiology
Upper extremity	Trauma
Humeral head	Corticosteroids
Capitellum	Sickle cell disease
Distal ulna	Alcoholism
Scaphoid	Gaucher's disease
Lunate	Nitrogen narcosis
Metacarpal head	Radiation
Phalanges	Collagen disease
Axial skeleton	Pancreatitis
Vertebral body[a]	Idiopathic
Iliac crest[a]	
Ischium[a]	
Symphysis[a]	
Lower extremity	
Femoral head[a]	
Greater trochanter[a]	
Femoral condyles[a]	
Tibial plateau[a]	
Patella[a]	
Distal tibia[a]	
Talus[a]	
Calcaneous[a]	
Metatarsals[a]	

[a] Areas easily examined with MR imaging.
Data from refs. 11, 12, 24.

lowing core decompression (28). Later stages of AVN do not respond to core decompression. In these patients, arthroplasty is the procedure of choice.

Early detection of osteonecrosis with imaging techniques has been challenging despite the use of isotope studies and computed tomography (CT) (2,4,5,7,13,14,16,17,21). The challenge is greatest in the hip, where early diagnosis is critical in planning treatment. Radiographs are often normal in early stages of the disease. Isotope studies have been useful in this regard; but, problems occur with this technique as well. The findings on isotope scan may be difficult to interpret during the early phases. Comparison with the opposite hip is often inaccurate because the disease is bilateral in up to 81% of patients (Table 2) (22).

Ficat (11) and Ficat and Arlet (12) described the stages of osteonecrosis of the femoral head based on radiographic features (Table 2). In stage 0 and I there are no radiographic findings. Radiographic findings are often subtle in stage II, especially early. Frog leg oblique views and tomography may be useful in this setting. The latter is especially helpful in differentiating stage II from early stage III (17). Diagnosis of stage III to IV is usually not difficult due to the prominent crescent sign and later articular collapse with joint space narrowing.

TABLE 2. *Staging of osteonecrosis*

Stage	Clinical	Radiograph	Isotope	MR imaging	Pathology
0	No symptoms	Normal	±	?	Hemopoietic and necrotic
I	May have symptoms	Normal or may have patchy osteoporosis	Uniform uptake	Signal intensity inhomogeneous	Sinus congestion, fibroblasts, hypoplastic marrow, empty lacunae
II	Pain, stiffness	Osteoporosis, mixed osteoporosis and sclerosis, cystic changes (may require tomography)	Nonuniform uptake	Wedge-shaped crescent sign (X-ray stage III)	Necrotic tissue, fatty tissue, margin fibrous with revascularization and new bone on dead trabeculae
III	Stiffness; groin and knee pain	Crescent sign, sequestra, cortical collapse, joint preserved	Photon deficient (cold spot)	Crescent sign, sequestra, cortical collapse, joint preserved	Necrosis surrounded by granulation tissue
IV	Pain and limp may be severe	III plus degenerative changes with narrowed joint space		III plus degenerative changes with narrowed joint space	Changes of III exaggerated

Data from ref. 6 and 11 to 13.

MR imaging shows great promise in early detection of AVN. Steinberg (23) studied 90 patients with suspected avascular necrosis of the hips. Biopsies were available in 55 of these patients. MR imaging was 96% accurate when compared with biopsy findings. Isotope studies and CT scans correlated with biopsy in 71 and 54%, respectively. The diagnosis was established earlier with MR imaging than with radiographs in 14 patients.

MR TECHNIQUES

MR studies for AVN can be accomplished quickly and easily. The lower extremity (Table 1) is examined using the corset or body coil (hips). The knees and ankles can be examined using the head coil to allow comparison of both sides. If necessary, surface coils can be used to confirm areas which are equivocal using the larger coils. Examination of the upper extremities is more difficult (see T. H. Berquist, "Technical Considerations in Magnetic Resonance Imaging," *this volume*). The body coil is often adequate for the shoulders, but surface coils

are needed for the elbow and wrist. Multislice coronal images using partial saturation technique (TE ≤ 30, TR ≤ 500) can be performed quickly (≤5 min).
The normal femoral head has uniformly high intensity (TE ≤ 30, TR 600) on
coronal images, except for the medial trabeculae of the femoral neck. This area
is seen as a lower intensity band extending into the femoral head (Fig. 1). If
findings are not obvious, axial or coronal multiecho (TE 25, 50, 75, 100; TR
2,000) images may show subtle changes not evident with the partial saturation
technique. To date the partial saturation sequences have usually been sufficient.
The involved area will have a low signal intensity margin with either normal or
inhomogeneous intensity in the subchondral bone (Fig. 2).

We have noted that MR imaging not only detects AVN of the hip more easily
than isotopes or radiographs, but, in addition, the stage of disease is more advanced than one would judge from radiographs (Table 2). When radiographs
are normal or show only sclerotic areas (stage II), MR images demonstrate changes
at the stage III level (Fig. 2). This may indicate the need for significant changes
in classification and the approach to treatment. In later stages of disease the MR
findings and radiographs correlate more closely (Fig. 2, right hip).

Detection of stage 0 and I with MR imaging is theoretically possible, but
current experience is too limited to determine the accuracy in detecting very
early changes or how early changes may present (Fig. 3). The MR signal in the
femoral head is due to fat and hemopoietic cells. Fat cells may remain viable
for up to 48 hr. Thus, when the number of fat cells diminishes, one might expect
the signal intensity to decrease (Fig. 2) (27). However, fat may remain in the
extracellular state, and the image appearance may not change significantly.

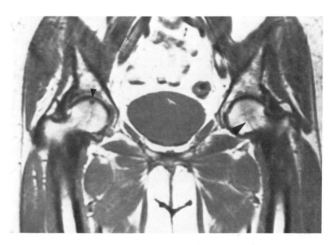

FIG. 1. Coronal image of the femoral heads (TE 25, TR 600). Note the low intensity trabecular
pattern now extending into the left femoral head (*arrow*). There is a well-marginated degenerative
cyst in the right hip (*arrow*).

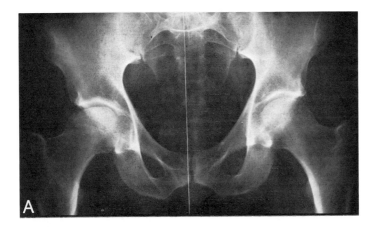

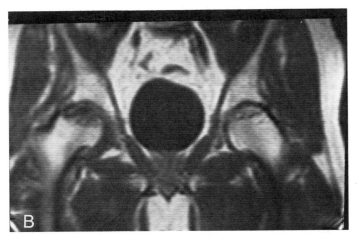

FIG. 2. Bilateral AVN of the femoral heads. **A:** Anteroposterior view of the pelvis shows advanced AVN on the right (stage IV) with no obvious abnormality on the left. **B:** Coronal partial saturation images of the hip show advanced AVN bilaterally. Changes on the left would coincide with stage III disease radiographically.

Chemical shift imaging or water–fat images may be helpful in evaluating early AVN.

The changes, especially early, are not specific for AVN. However, MR studies are very useful in characterizing AVN and in identifying other conditions which present with pain and may mimic avascular necrosis.

The patient in Fig. 4 presented with hip pain and was suspected of having avascular necrosis. Radiographs were normal, but MR images showed decreased signal in the femoral head and upper femur, consistent with transient osteoporosis of the hip. This finding would not be confused with AVN. Other conditions

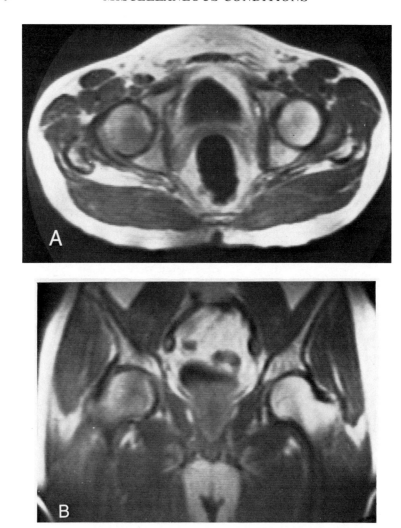

FIG. 3. Early AVN of the right femoral head. There is decreased signal intensity in the anterior portion of the right femoral head on the partial saturation axial **(A)** and coronal views **(B)**. Stage I.

presenting with pain can be differentiated from AVN using MR imaging (Figs. 1 and 5).

Although work is still in progress, it is clear that MR imaging is very effective in early detection of avascular necrosis. Further research is needed to define the early image characteristics and role of spectroscopy in detecting stage 0 and I disease.

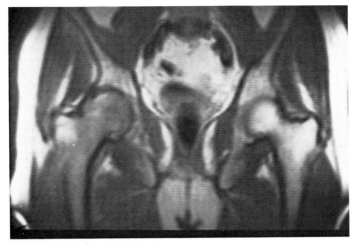

FIG. 4. MR on patient with transient osteoporosis of the hip. There is decreased signal in the femoral head, neck, and upper femur (TE 30, TR 500). Findings are not characteristic of osteonecrosis.

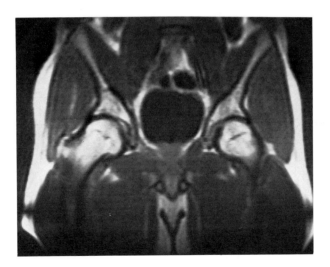

FIG. 5. Young patient with hip pain. The coronal partial saturation images (TE 30, TR 500) **(A)** show thickening of the ligamentum teres (*arrow*) which was causing clicking and locking of the hip.

MYOPATHIES

The MR characteristics of soft tissue infection, trauma and neoplasm are discussed elsewhere (T. H. Berquist, "Bone and Soft Tissue Tumors;" T. H. Berquist, "Musculoskeletal Infection;" T. H. Berquist, R. L. Ehman, J. A. Rand, and S. Scott "Musculoskeletal Trauma"). Early experience suggests MR imaging may also play a significant role in evaluation of other primary muscle and neuromuscular disorders. Both imaging and spectroscopy will be valuable in this regard (1,9,10,15,17,20,25).

IMAGING

Current imaging techniques provide limited information about nonneoplastic muscle diseases. Routine radiographic techniques are of little value even with low kilovoltage or xerox techniques. Several authors have studied computed tomographic features of myopathies (15,17,25). O'Doherty et al. (17) described patterns of muscle replacement using CT. Both localized and diffuse low-density areas were noted in patients with pseudohypertrophic muscular dystrophy. Changes in selected muscle groups have been reported in Duchenne's muscular dystrophy (15). Hawley et al. (15) demonstrated that CT scans of patients with neuromuscular diseases initially showed atrophy of muscles followed by decreased muscle density. Primary myopathies revealed similar changes but in reverse order with decreased density preceding muscle atrophy. The low density areas in muscle seen on CT are likely due to fat and/or connective tissue replacement. Termote et al. (25) noted that these fat cells are smaller than normal, so in early stages of the disease the muscle volume may appear normal clinically. Thus early detection with MR imaging can provide valuable clinical information.

MR imaging has soft tissue contrast superior to CT. Therefore, detection of early muscle changes can be more easily accomplished. From an imaging standpoint the findings seen on MR imaging may be no more specific than CT. However, certain important changes can be noted with MR. The muscle groups can be easily distinguished, and the extent of involvement determined by using multiple image planes (Fig. 6). Using both T1- and T2-weighted images, it is possible to distinguish early edema or inflammation (white on T2- and black on T1-weighted images) (Fig. 7) from fatty infiltration or replacement (Fig. 8). Fatty infiltration will have high signal intensity (white) on both T1- and T2-weighted sequences. Acute hemorrhage may be confused with edema. A history of trauma and sequential changes of hemorrhage are useful in differentiating parenchymal hemorrhage from edema. Further refinement can be accomplished using chemical shift imaging. This allows differentiation of signal emitted from fat and water. The technique may also be useful in evaluating certain storage diseases (20).

Borghi et al. (1) also studied T1 relaxation times. They noted that T1 relaxation times were considerably reduced in patients with myopathy (normal 450 to 800

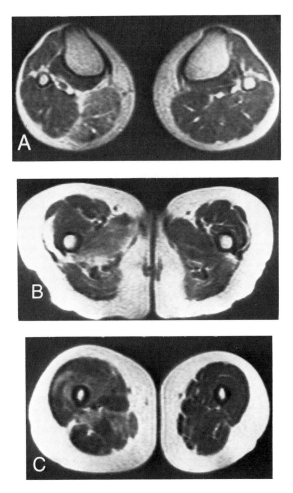

FIG. 6. Myopathy. **A:** Axial T2-weighted images show an infiltrative inflammatory process involving only the medial gastrocnemius. **B, C:** Axial T2-weighted images of the thighs in a patient with nodular polymyositis. There is diffuse muscle involvement.

msec, myopathy ≤ 500 msec). This is undoubtedly due to replacement of muscle with fat and fibrous tissue. Although further studies are needed, these data may be useful in differentiating myopathy from other pathology such as neoplasm, where T1 values are elevated.

The potential imaging role of MR imaging in evaluating myopathies includes the following: (a) clearly defining the muscle groups involved, (b) differentiating atrophy and fatty replacement from more acute inflammatory changes, (c) following treatment phases and progression of disease, and (d) localizing optimal sites for biopsy. Current use of imaging parameters alone does not obviate the

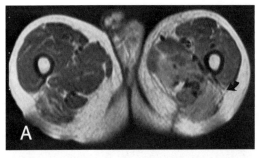

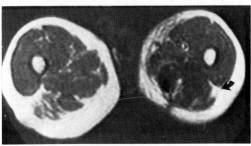

FIG. 7. Muscle inflammation with edema and hemorrhage. Edema with its high water content has long T1 and T2 relaxation times. The T2-weighted image (**A**) (TE 60, TR 2,000) shows a high-intensity infiltrative process. The T1-weighted image (IR 500/2,000) (**B**) shows the abnormality is low intensity. This allows differentiation from fatty infiltration (*arrows*) at the margin of the edema and hemorrhage.

need for clinical and histochemical studies to completely define the pathologic process.

SPECTROSCOPY

The ability to evaluate nuclei other than hydrogen adds to the potential role of MR imaging for evaluation of myopathies. With higher magnetic fields, imaging and spectropic studies (^{31}P, ^{23}Na, ^{13}C, and other nuclei) may be possible. Individual peaks of ATP (adenosine triphosphate) can be identified spectroscopically. ^{31}P studies may be helpful for monitoring drug therapy and evaluating patients with metabolic disorders and muscular storage diseases. For example, nuclear magnetic resonance (NMR) ^{31}P spectroscopy has shown a decrease in total phosphorus in patients with muscular dystrophy (10).

The optimal field strength for chemical work has not yet been determined. Further research and clinical trials will be required before the role of spectroscopy is completely understood.

ARTICULAR DISORDERS

The role of MR imaging in trauma, infection, and neoplastic disorders of the joints has been discussed elsewhere (T. H. Berquist, "Bone and Soft Tissue Tumors;" T. H. Berquist, "Musculoskeletal Infection;" and T. H. Berquist et al., "Musculoskeletal Trauma"). However, other inflammatory arthritides deserve

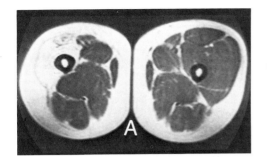

FIG. 8. Fatty replacement due to chronic neuropathy. The axial T2-weighted image (TE 60, TR 2,000) (**A**) and coronal partial saturation image (**B**) show complete fatty replacement of the muscle. The fatty tissue maintains its high signal intensity on both sequences.

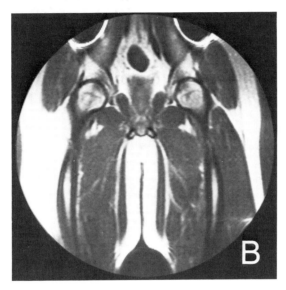

mention. Currently, diagnosis of rheumatoid and other types of arthritis is based on laboratory studies, clinical data, and radiographic techniques (radiographs, xerograms, magnification technique) (26). Soft tissue changes occur prior to bony erosion and articular destruction. The superior soft tissue contrast of MR may, therefore, provide detection of soft tissue changes earlier than other conventional techniques. Animal studies demonstrate that inflammatory joint changes can be identified by increased signal intensity on T2-weighted (TE 60, TR 2,000) sequences. Relaxation times (T1 and T2) are also increased (26). Detection of bone changes and fluid in the joint capsule may also be possible during the early stages of disease when radiographs are normal (Fig. 9).

These changes may not allow the specific type of arthritis to be diagnosed. However, coupled with clinical and laboratory studies arthritis may be detected earlier.

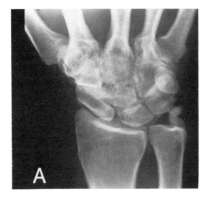
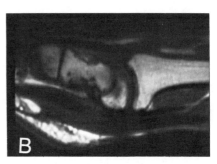

FIG. 9. Patient with chronic wrist pain. **A:** Arthrogram shows contrast in the distal radioulnar and intercarpal compartments. The bones are normal. **B:** Sagittal MR image (TE 25, TR 500) shows volar subluxation of the lunate with an area of necrosis (low intensity) in the distal articular portion. There are also numerous erosions in the capitate.

Certain joints may be particularly suited to MR examinations. For example, the temporomandibular joint (TMJ) is often difficult to evaluate. Tomography and arthrography are commonly used. However, surface coil MR images provide excellent detail of the articular surface and disk (19). Although experience is limited thus far, in the future MR may obviate the need for arthrography (Fig. 10).

Deformity of joints, especially in the spine, in patients with rheumatoid arthritis may lead to significant complications. MR imaging is ideally suited for evaluating the relationship of vertebrae, brainstem, and clivus (Fig. 11).

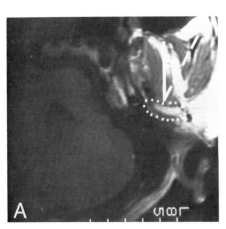
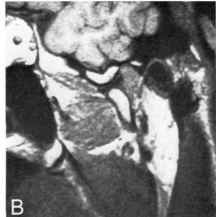

FIG. 10. Normal TMJ (1.5 T, TE 25, TR 500). **A:** The patient should be obliqued slightly to align the joint for sagittal surface coil images. **B:** Sagittal view of the normal TMJ.

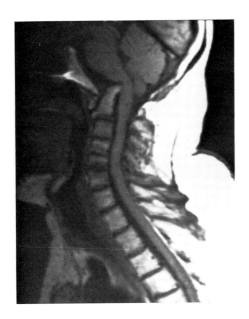

FIG. 11. Sagittal MR image of the upper cervical spine (TE 30, TR 500; 1.5 T, surface coil) in a patient with rheumatoid arthritis. There is upward displacement of the odontoid with marked deviation and slight anterior compression of the cord. There is also compression of several vertebrae (C4 to C6).

BONE MARROW DISORDERS

Bone marrow changes normally with age and may be affected by malignant (see T. H. Berquist, "Bone and Soft Tissue Tumors," *this volume*), inflammatory, and other infiltrative processes. The distribution of trabecular bone, fat, and hematopoietic tissues change normally with age (6). Mineral content decreases with age, especially in women after menopause. There is also a decrease in red marrow and an increase in fatty marrow with age. Reports indicate that T1 and T2 relaxation times also decrease with age. MR images show subtle but definite change with age (Fig. 12).

Pathologic processes in marrow result in increased signal intensity on T2-weighted sequences and areas of decreased intensity when partial saturation sequences are used. These findings are not specific and have been described with leukemia, certain anemias, and Gaucher's disease (Fig. 13) (3,6). Despite this lack of specificity MR is still useful in early detection of marrow abnormalities and allows one to choose appropriate biopsy sites. In addition response to treatment can also be evaluated. Changes in the marrow can be followed, and, for example if steroids are used in treatment, MR can be useful in differentiating pain due to progression of disease from osteonecrosis (Fig. 14).

CONGENITAL DISORDERS

Routine radiographs will continue to play a major role in identification of congenital disorders. MR offers several potential advantages for study of con-

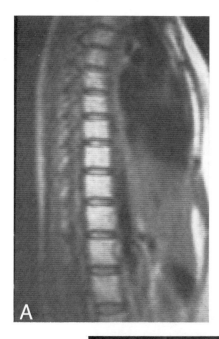

FIG. 12. Normal sagittal MR images of the spine (TE 30, TR 500). **A:** 18 year old female. The signal intensity of the vertebral marrow and discs is nearly equal. **B:** 67 year old female. The signal intensity is decreased in the vertebrae. Note the localized areas of increased intensity, presumably due to intravertebral fat collections.

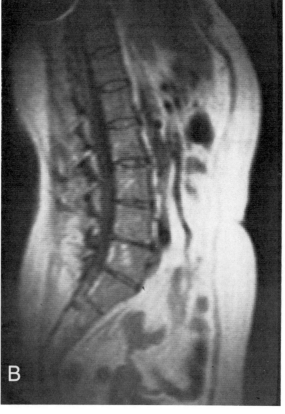

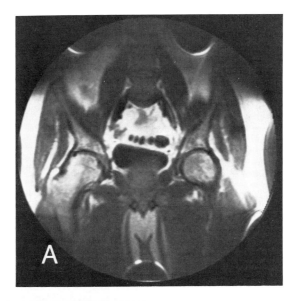

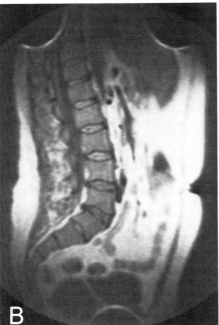

FIG. 13. Gaucher's disease. Coronal images of the pelvis (**A**) and sagittal images of the spine (**B**) show diffuse decrease in signal intensity (TE 30, TR 500; 0.15 T).

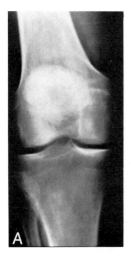
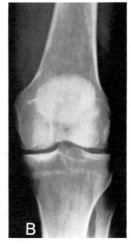

FIG. 14.   Patient with lymphoma and knee pain. Radiographs (**A,B**) are normal. Coronal MR images of both knees (**C**) and the left knee (**D**) demonstrate osteonecrosis in the articular surfaces of the tibias and femurs and bone infarcts bilaterally due to steroid therapy (TE 30, TR 500).

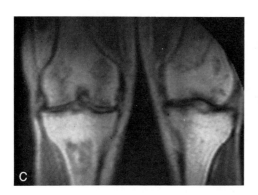
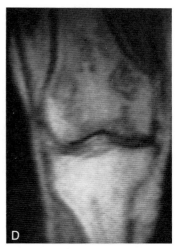

genital hip disease, tibial torsion, and certain bone formation disorders. There is no ionizing radiation with MR. Images of the extremities can be obtained in the axial plane providing measurement capabilities similiar to those used in CT. Sagittal and coronal images may provide additional information. Depending on the patient's age, unossified ossification centers can also be identified which may provide earlier evaluation of growth disturbances and other abnormalities (Fig. 15).

PITFALLS AND NORMAL VARIANTS

Errors in interpretation can occur with any imaging technique. Complex anatomy is clearly demonstrated with MR, especially using the coronal and sagittal

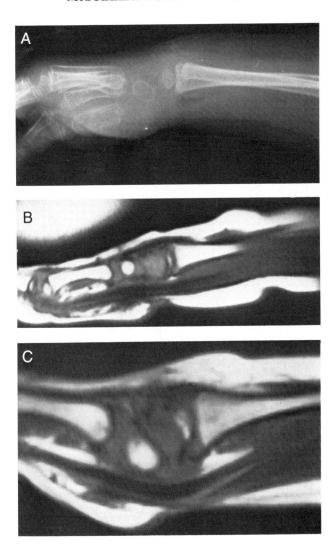

FIG. 15. Three year old with pain and function loss in the wrist. **A:** Lateral radiographs showing incomplete ossification of the carpal bones. Sagittal MR images (TE 25, TR 500) of the normal (**B**) and abnormal wrist (**C**) show that there is carpal collapse with shortening in the involved wrist.

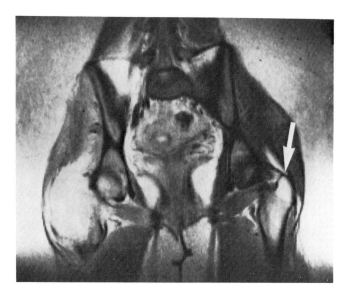

FIG. 16. High intensity signal from normal apophysis. This coronal image of a 28 year old woman with a giant cell tumor in the right hip shows the high intensity signal often seen in normal epiphyses and apophyses (*arrow*) in young adults and children.

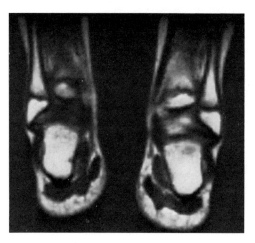

FIG. 17. High intensity signal from normal apophysis. This coronal image of the ankles in this child shows the normal high intensity which can occur in the apophyses in children.

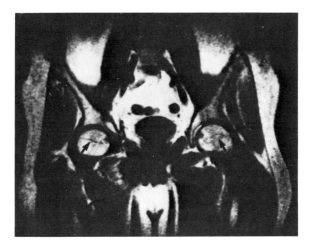

FIG. 18. Epiphyseal remnant. A coronal scan through the pelvis shows a linear area of low intensity signal in the femoral heads (*arrows*). These are the normal physeal lines and should not be confused with fractures.

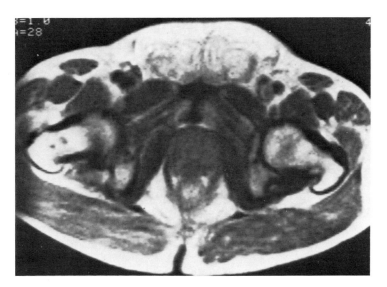

FIG. 19. Fibrous cortical defects or herniation pits in the femoral neck. An axial image through the hips shows two low-intensity signal areas in the right femoral neck which represent either fibrous cortical defects or benign herniation pits of the femoral neck. These should not be confused with metastatic disease.

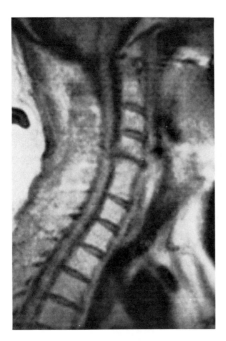

FIG. 20. Sagittal T1-weighted (TR/TE of 600/ 40 msec, 0.15 T) image of the cervical spine in a 62 year old male with a congenital block vertebra at the C5–6 level. The intervertebral disc space at C4–5 is narrowed and has decreased intensity, consistent with degenerative disc disease. Also shown at this level is posterior osteophytosis, causing some compromise of the anteroposterior diameter of the cervical canal.

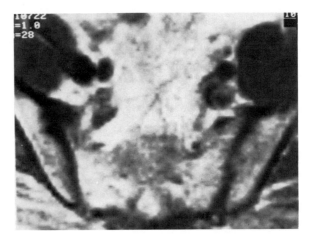

FIG. 21. SI joint sclerosis. A coronal scan through the sacroiliac joints shows low-intensity signal in the anterior portion of the right SI joint involving both the sacral and iliac sides of the joint. This is typical of degenerative disease involving the SI joint; however, a spondyloarthropathy such as psoriatic disease or Reiter's and even infection could certainly present with this appearance.

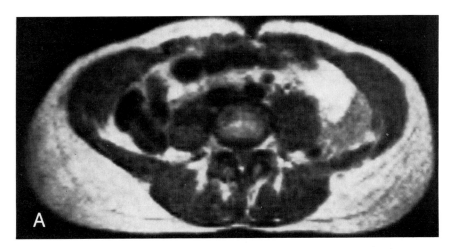

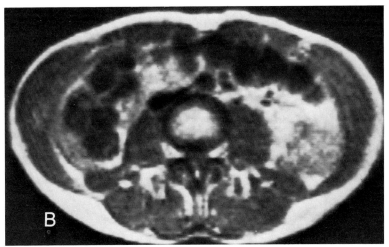

FIG. 22. Loss of disc signal from partial volume averaging. **A:** A scan through the disc of the lumbar spine shows a low intensity signal of the disc material which is consistent with degenerative disc disease. However, the adjacent slice shown in **B** shows the disc to have the normal high-intensity signal. Slice **A** shows the disc to be low intensity signal because of partial volume averaging with the end-plate.

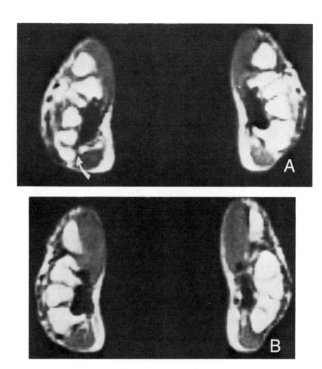

FIG. 23. Partial volume averaging of the hamate simulating a fracture. **A:** Axial scan of the wrist with an apparent fracture (*arrow*) of the hook of the hamate on the right side. Compare this with the normal hook of the hamate on the left side. **B:** The adjacent slice, however, shows the hook of the hamate on the right to be normal. The apparent fracture in **A** is due to partial volume averaging.

planes. Therefore, it is essential that clinicians and imagers be familiar with normal anatomy and variants so errors in interpretation can be avoided. Although MR is still being evaluated, many of these potential problems can be avoided by using knowledge gained with CT and radiographs where more experience with normal variants has been obtained (18). Compared to more conventional techniques, many variants have a similar appearance on MR images (Figs. 16 to 21).

Additional problems in interpretation may occur due to partial volume effects (Figs. 22 to 24). This problem is well known due to our previous experience with CT.

Other considerations include improper choice of pulse sequence (Fig. 25), chemical shift artifact, and other artifacts due to problems with software or hardware. Chemical shift artifacts are particularly troublesome at the boundaries of normal anatomic structures and can result in distortion of the anatomy or confusing normal structures with pathology. The artifact is usually paired and consistent and changes orientation when the direction of frequency encoding is

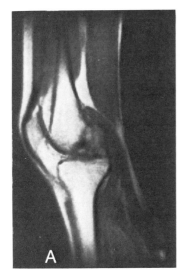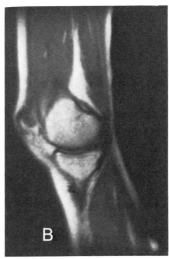

FIG. 24. Partial volume averaging in the knee simulating cortical destruction. **A:** Irregularity and apparent cortical destruction of the posterior part of the epicondyle in the femur. **B:** The adjacent slice, however, shows the cortex to be intact. The irregularity and apparent cortical destruction of the cortex in **A** is due to partial volume averaging in the region of the intercondylar notch.

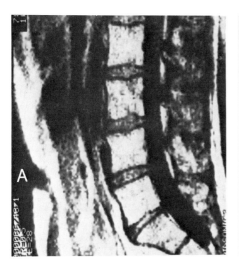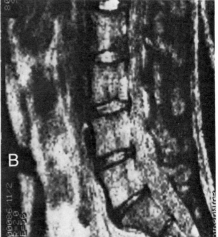

FIG. 25. A: Sagittal T1-weighted (TR/TE of 500/28 msec, 0.35 T) image of a normal lumbosacral spine. With these parameters it is difficult to distinguish the posterior annular fibers from the thecal contents. **B:** Sagittal T2-weighted (TR/TE of 2,000/56 msec, 0.35 T) image of the same spine. The interface between the posterior disc margins and the thecal contents is now much easier to evaluate.

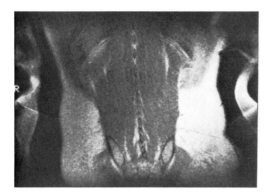

FIG. 26. Intensity artifact. A coronal scan through the back shows an artifact of the image being darker on one side than the other. Note the high intensity signal from the muscles on the left as compared to the right. The exact cause of this is undetermined. Note also the distortion of the arms which is due to patient contact with the coils.

changed (8). There are still artifacts and variations in image intensity which are not completely understood (Fig. 26). As experience increases many of these problems will be solved, increasing the confidence and accuracy of image interpretation.

REFERENCES

1. Borghi, L., Savoldi, F., Scelsi, R., and Villa, M. (1983): Nuclear magnetic resonance response of protons in normal and pathologic muscles. *Exp. Neurol.,* 81:89–96.
2. Caballero-Carpena, O., and Pardo-Montaner, J. (1983): Contribution to the diagnoses of idiopathic femoral head necrosis by scintigraphy with ^{99}TC-MDP assessed quantitatively by computer. *Nucl. Med.,* 22:232–236.
3. Cohen, M. D., Klatte, E. C., Boehner, R., Smith, J. A., Martin-Simmerman, P., Carr, B. E., Provisor, A. T., Weetman, B. M., Coates, T., Siddiqui, A., Weiseman, S. J., Berkow, R., McKenna, S., and McGuire, W. A. (1984): Magnetic resonance imaging of bone marrow disease in children. *Radiology,* 151:715–718.
4. Dihlmann, W. (1982): CT analyses of the upper end of the femur: The asterisk sign of ischemic bone necrosis of the femoral head. *Skeletal Radiol.,* 8:251–258.
5. Dodig, D., Ugarkovic, B., and Orlic, D. (1983): Bone scintigraphy in idiopathic aseptic femoral head necrosis. *Eur. J. Nucl. Med.,* 8:23–25.
6. Dooms, G. C., Fisher, M. R., Hricak, H., Richardson, M., Crook, L. F., and Genant, H. K. (1985): Bone marrow imaging: Magnetic resonance studies related to age and sex. *Radiology,* 155:429–432.
7. Drane, W. E., and Rudd, T. G. (1985): Femoral head viability following hip fracture. *Clin. Nucl. Med.,* 10:141–146.
8. Dwyer, A. J., Knop, R. H., and Hoult, D. I. (1985): Frequency shift artifacts in MR imaging. *J. Comput. Assist. Tomogr.,* 9:16–18.
9. Edwards, R. H. T., Dawson, M. J., Griffith, J. R., Gorton, R., and Wilk, C. (1983): Nuclear magnetic resonance spectroscopy in research and clinical diagnosis. *Eur. J. Clin. Invest.,* 13:429–431.
10. Edwards, R. H. T., Dawson, M. J., Wilkie, R. E., and Shaw, D. (1982): Clinical use of nuclear magnetic resonance in investigation of myopathy. *Lancet,* 1:725–731.
11. Ficat, R. F. (1983): Treatment of avascular necrosis of the femoral head. *Hip,* 2:279–295.
12. Ficat, R. F., and Arlet, J. (1980): *Ischemia and Necrosis of Bone,* edited by D. S. Hungerford. Williams and Wilkens, Baltimore.
13. Greiff, J., Lang, S., Hoilund-Carlsen, P. F., Karle, A. K., and Uhrenholdt, A. (1980): Early detection of ^{99}TC-SN-pyrophosphate scintigraphy of femoral head necrosis following medial femoral neck fractures. *Acta Orthop. Scand.,* 51:119–125.

14. Greyson, N. D., Lotem, M. M., Gross, A. E., and Houpt, J. B. (1982): Radionuclide evaluation of spontaneous femoral osteonecrosis. *Radiology,* 142:729–735.
15. Hawley, R. J., Schllinger, D., and O'Doherty, D. S. (1984): Computed tomographic patterns of muscle in neuromuscular diseases. *Arch. Neurol.,* 41:383–387.
16. Lucie, R. S., Fuller, S., Burdick, D. C., and Johnston, R. M. (1980): Early prediction of avascular necrosis of the femoral head following femoral neck fractures. *Clin. Orthop.,* 161:207–214.
17. O'Doherty, D. S., Schellinger, D., and Raptopoulos, V. (1977): Computed tomographic patterns of pseudohypertrophic muscular dystrophy: Preliminary results. *J. Comput. Assist. Tomogr.,* 14: 482–486.
18. Pitt, M. J., Graham, A. R., Shipman, J. H., and Birkby, W. L. (1982): Herniation pit of the femoral neck. *A. J. R.,* 138:1115–1121.
19. Roberts, D., Schenck, J., Joseph, P., Foster, T., Hart, H., Pettigrew, J., Keindel, H. L., Edelstein, W., and Haber, B. (1985): Temporomandibular joint: Magnetic resonance imaging. *Radiology,* 155:829–830.
20. Scott, J. A., Rosenthal, D. I., and Brady, T. J. (1984): The evaluation of musculoskeletal disease with magnetic resonance imaging. *Radiol. Clin. North Am.,* 22:917–924.
21. Soles, P. V., Yoon, Y. S., Makley, J. T., and Kalamchi, A. (1984): Nuclear magnetic resonance imaging in Legg–Calve–Perthes Disease. *J. Bone Joint Surg. [Am.],* 66:1357–1363.
22. Springfield, D. S., and Ennelung, W. J. (1978): Surgery for aseptic necrosis of the femoral head. *Clin. Orthop.,* 130:175–178.
23. Steinberg, M. (1985): MRI in avascular necrosis of the femoral head. *Ann. Meet. Am. Acad. Orthoped. Surgeons, 52nd, Las Vegas, Nevada, Feb., 1985.*
24. Sweet, D. E., and Madewell, J. E. (1981): Pathogenesis of osteonecrosis. In: *Diagnosis of Bone and Joint Disorders,* edited by D. Resnick and G. Niewayama, pp. 2780–2871. W.B. Saunders, Philadelphia.
25. Termote, J., Baert, A., Crolla, D., Palmers, Y., and Bulcke, J. A. (1980): Computed tomography of the normal and pathologic muscular system. *Radiology,* 137:439–444.
26. Terrier, F., Hricak, H., Revel, D., Alpers, C. E., Reinhold, C. E., Levine, J., and Genant, H. K. (1985): Magnetic resonance imaging and spectroscopy of periarticular inflammatory soft tissue changes in experimental arthritis of the rat. *Invest. Radiol.,* 20:813–823.
27. Totty, W. G., Murphy, W. A., Ganz, W. I., Kumar, B., Davin, W. J., and Siegel, B. A. (1984): Magnetic resonance imaging of the normal and ischemic femoral head. *A. J. R.,* 143:1273–1280.
28. Wang, G. J., Dughman, S. S., Reger, S. I., and Stamp, W. G. (1985): The effect of core decompression on femoral head blood flow in steroid-induced avascular necroses of the femoral head. *J. Bone Joint Surg. [Am.],* 67A:121–124.

Subject Index

Subject Index

A

Abscess, differential diagnosis, 102,103
Achilles tendon, 156,157,158
  tear, 150–159,160
Acquisition time, defined, 17
Adductor tear, 139
Air, signal intensity, 166–167
Anatomy, normal, variants, 200–208
Anemia, 178
Aneurysm clip, 69
Ankle, 158–159
  arteriovenous malformation, 94
Annulus
  anterior, 165,166
  posterior, 165,166
Aorta, descending, 61
Apophysis, normal, 202
Arteriovenous malformation, 94
Artery. *See specific type*
Arthritis, 195,196,197
  infectious, 114–116
Arthrography
  knee, 140,142
  subtraction, 118
Arthroscopy, knee, 140–141,142
Articular disorder, 194–196
Artifact, 65–66,69–71
  beam-hardening, 85,87
  chemical shift, 206–208
  clip, 98,99
  infection, 118–120
  intensity, 208
  motion, 42
  nonferromagnetic material, 69–71
  tumor recurrence evaluation, 106
Atherosclerosis, 55
Axial plane, spine, 165

B

B_0, defined, 17
B_1, defined, 17
Blood flow
  cutoff velocity, 62

flow related enhancement, 56,57
  saturation, 56,57
  spin dephasing effect, 56–61
  washout effects, 56,61–62
Blood vessel, signal intensity, 65–66
Bone
  lymphoma, 99,100
  relaxation time, 31–32
Bone infarct
  etiology, 186
  site, 186
Bone lesion, benign, 99
Bone marrow disorder, 197
Brownian jump, 28
Bulk magnetization, 27
  vector, 27
Bursa, 156
Bursitis, 128

C

Calcification, 99,100,101
Calf muscle, 156
Cardiac monitoring, 68
  equipment, 68
Cartilage
  articular, signal intensity, 65–66
  menical, signal intensity, 65
Cast, 70
Cerebrospinal fluid, 167–168
Chemical shift
  artifact, 206–208
  defined, 17
  resonant frequency, 27
  techniques, 52,53–55
Chemonucleolysis, 179–180,181
Chondrosarcoma, 101
Chymopapain, 180,181
Claustrophobia, 66–68
Clip, 69
Coil
  body, 70,76
  coupled, 70,75,76
  defined, 17